WITHDRAWN

PAYING *the* PRICE

D0543076

Dedication

This book was written originally for my family Mum, Dad, Paul, Kristy, Nicholas to tell them why I kept on crying but really it is for everybody who has helped me grow strong and who has inspired me to be the person I am today. Special thanks to my husband Adrian Millward-McHugh who was the reason I started fighting back. My Mum Linda Millward was so strong and heroic throughout my journey and I can't thank her enough for the endless ways she lifted me up every time I was knocked down. Thank you Mum for everything!

About Stephanie Millward

Stephanie Millward has lived three different lives. The first a perfect one full of dreams and ambitions. This one had to die and was replaced by a sorrowful battle against Multiple Sclerosis then the third is full of hope and inspiration proving that a dream can be all the strength you need to pull yourself out of a dark hole.

Stephanie's story is not about a girl who lost her career, her health, her Dad, her dog and her friend but instead is about a young lady who was walking through a dark tunnel, eventually reaching the light at the end and meeting her guardian angel, her partner for life - the fairytale story. Her story is a little harsher than the fairy stories but it is still about reaching all the goals of the younger girl and even of realising all her dreams. It is a story about hope and about inspiration even through the dark times. It is a book about becoming the person you have always dreamed about. A shattered perfection rebuilt to enable the light to reflect again. The end to one of those stunning rainbows.

PAYING *the* PRICE

Stephanie Millward

BROWN
DOG
BOOKS

Published under licence by Brown Dog Books and The Self Publishing Partnership
7 Green Park Station, Bath BA1 1JB

www.selfpublishingpartnership.co.uk

ISBN Printed book: 978-1-903056-79-0
ISBN E-book: 978-1-903056-86-8

Cover design by Kevin Rylands

Printed and bound by CPI Group (UK) Ltd, Croydon CR0 4YY

CONTENTS

CHAPTER 1

Paying the Price

Crying floods of tears, I start writing. The pain inside my heart screaming silent words of loss, loneliness, fear. What have I done wrong? I don't deserve this. Why is it getting me now? It's so dark and terrifying. Why me?

Waking the next morning I see my notebook with the words of my poem etched neatly inside. Wondering what I had written I pulled the book closer.

'Paying the Price.'

The title was printed darker than the other words as though the pain was being pushed through the paper. The three words seemed so perfect for the pain I was feeling at that moment, especially the immense pain down the whole of my left side which felt to me like my body is trying to expand and get out but the skin is too thin and fragile, and definitely far too small, but still managing to hold it all in. Paying for something I must have done wrong and the price being the rest of my life. The doctors had just diagnosed me as suffering from Multiple Sclerosis (MS), a disease of the central nervous system (the brain and spinal cord). With no known cure and the doctors seemingly nowhere near the cure, I was so scared. What will happen to me now?

I had been living such a perfect life with everything going exactly the way I had dreamed: winning medals every time I swam; getting straight A grades at school without any revision; my friends at school saying I had perfect parents; never at the doctors; perfect eyesight and no fillings! I was living the perfect life. Why did it all have to change? Why did everything have to end? Why did I have to get sick?

My eyesight was the first thing to be hit. My 20/20 vision disappeared and it was replaced by unfocussed colours and a continuous bouncing: one eye jumping left to right and the other going up and down, both of which left of me tripping and wobbling as though I had drunk far too much! 'Why does my vision have to keep moving? Why can't it stop? I can't focus on anything with all the movement. Please make it stop.' I had asked the doctors this many times but they had just looked right through me as they often do. 'An incurable illness,' they had said, as if that was the only answer. An incurable illness? Are they even looking for a cure at the moment or is this something that will remain 'incurable' forever?

Does this mean that there is no point me being alive now as even the doctors can't help me? Maybe I should just end the pain now. I have let everyone down any way, nobody would notice if I wasn't here. 'There's nothing I can do'? The doctor's voice ringing in my ears 'There's nothing I can do.'

Looking for a way to stop my eyes from jumping I turn to lie down – no, that just causes the dizzy feeling and a powerful sense of nausea. Shut one eye? - yeah that helps a little. Reading on, I see I have written in my diary: 'Why are we waiting? What are we waiting for?' This was referring to the drug Beta Interferon that Wiltshire's Health Authority are not funding for the sufferers of Multiple Sclerosis who live in Wiltshire, just because of where they live. Interesting! I am sure this country has a '*National* Health Service?'

Hearing a small noise from outside my room I move and open the door to allow my little Yorkshire terrier, Spring, to run inside yapping, licking and kissing. Spring always gives me the merriest welcome with her wagging stump of a tail and all her excitement. I kiss her back feeling her warmth beneath my arms. I read the poem to Spring and she just looked at me with loving eyes as a mother would to her child. She obviously liked the poem! It made me cry yet again to hear my own words. Spring just moved closer to me - protecting.

I decided to send the poem to be printed in the local paper the *Bath Chronicle*, to show other people how much I was hurting so that maybe someone could take my pain away. It was printed the next day - my whole letter as though the editor needed to show all my naked feelings, I cried again. The picture of me in the paper didn't look good; it looked as though my eyes were crying and my brain was alive but almost ready to explode with the pain. I look back at this picture now and I see just the size of my huge broken heart. An amazing life with incredible dreams, all ripped away like an old poster torn from the wall and then discarded like rubbish. An amazing sixteen years stopped in mid-flow and replaced by a dungeon, a black hole engulfing me, surrounding me completely and dragging me down... down... down.

To Whom It May Concern,

My name is Stephanie Millward. The *Bath Chronicle* has represented my case many times. My story is well known to anyone who reads the *Bath Chronicle* and so I have decided to send this poem to be printed.

I have Multiple Sclerosis. With the help of the newspaper I was given the chance to try a drug that tries to stabilise MS. I was given the drug on a trial basis and so I am in the process of waiting for the National Institute of Clinical Excellence (NICE) to make a decision on the cost effectiveness of the drug.

I was crying floods of tears when I wrote this poem. It relates all of my fears in a few small words. I wish that the NICE would listen to these small words and help me out.

NICE - Please help us

Paying the Price

Why are we waiting?
What are we waiting for?
Will the drug fix our problems?
Will it defeat the MS War?

Why are we fighting?
What are we fighting for?
Is it the needles? Is it more pain?
Why are we fighting? It's not a game.

I'm paying the price,
Paying it every day.
Holding onto memories,
Grasping in every way.

Keep a smile on your face,
Make it all look fine.
Speak with no disgrace,
Hide the hurt inside.

I try not to quit,
I try not to cry.
Parts of me hurting,
Parts wanting to die.

Why are we waiting?
Why can't we dance?
We're only human,
Please give us a chance.

Stephanie Millward Copyright 2000

Please would you to print this as it may show the hurt and the pain that all MS sufferers are going through with regards to the drug Beta Interferon.

The line 'Why can't we dance?' has many hidden reasons. I am 19 years old. Most other 19 year old teenagers spend Saturday night out at the clubs or pubs; I spend mine in front of a television set because I can't dance or drink alcohol safely. Many other MS sufferers can't dance because their condition has deteriorated so much. Another reason for writing it is that people normally dance or sing when they are happy. MS sufferers are not happy with NICE because they are not giving us a chance to live our lives normally.

Thank you, for everything.

Yours sincerely,
Stephanie Millward

I was definitely paying the price with the almost continual pain in my arms and legs (a side effect of MS) but I'm still not certain what I have done wrong or whether it will get any better in time. Probably not. I thought 'Paying the Price' was a wonderful name for my poem. A definite exclamation of life with no hope; a payment that will never end and a price that, for me, will probably be forever increasing.

CHAPTER 2
The Road to Work

Putting the paper away I start dressing for work. The local Co-operative just up the road was a perfect place because it was only a five minute walk away and I got to see my work friends every day.

I kiss Spring goodbye and start the familiar walk knowing it will be difficult today. A sharp pain has already spread down my left leg accompanied by a numbing pain in my left wrist; the familiar MS pains, and I know there are no ways to ease them. No paracetamol or ibuprofen tablets work to dull the pains; I just have to try to ignore them.

Reaching a total distance of just twenty metres, literally dragging my legs over the road, I stop knowing I won't be able to go any further. In my mind I question why there aren't any helpers or a lift or escalator up this hill. These may help hundreds of people, I am sure, but really they would help me now at this moment. Anything, anything would help me now.

I cry again out of complete frustration. It is only a short distance so I must be able to do it. I used to be able to, why can't I now? Why did it all have to end? Why did I have to get sick? I did everything right, I don't deserve this.

I try again. The right leg is stronger: start with that one.

'Forward,' I instruct. 'Move.'

Getting louder I start screaming at myself. Nothing happens and the legs keep up their ignorance. A bird in the sky chirps as if to tell me that shouting will not help.

'MOVE!' Nothing happens again and I fall to the road, crushed.

Pulling my phone out of my bag, I feel that I have lost again. Me against the MS and the MS is definitely the stronger one. Will it always be the stronger one? Will I be stuck asking mum for help every day?

My mum pulls up in her car. Seeing the look of concern in her eyes I tense, fearing the tears that may arrive if I say the wrong thing or if she asks the wrong question. I put my barriers up. I can't cry again, not yet.

'Do you want to go home or to work?' my mum asks.

'Work! Work! Definitely work!' I feel that if I get to work at least I would have almost beaten the MS, as it hasn't destroyed my whole day, yet!

Work cheered me up with all the same people coming in to say 'Hello' and to get their daily shopping. Each with a smile on their face. Each with a story of their own. Can they see my pain? Is it obvious with my covering smile? Have I got MS written all over my face?

'Keep working hard. Keep the MS away,' I tell myself. 'Please, keep it away. I am winning now. I am in charge.' It seemed so unfair that a teenager should have to put up with such a huge pressure of having an illness for the rest of her life. Wondering if the MS will get worse as it seems to be doing, or if I will need a wheelchair soon. Will I ever get married? Can anyone ever love me with this illness? It all seems so unfair, so incorrect. I am paying the price but what on earth did I do wrong? I have always been such a nice person, helping everybody out whenever I could. I have never been in detention at school and never got into a fight. Why did I get this illness? I didn't do anything wrong. I don't deserve this.

Why is it that 'only the good die young' as the saying goes? Why did I get sick as a child? Why is it that we find out about all the bad things that the good or famous people do as opposed to all the good things that they have done? Why, as a race, are we so pessimistic, and why do bad things seem to far outweigh the good things?

If I had been a bad person with spite and anger in my life would I have got MS? If I had been a couch potato watching television all day as opposed to swimming every day would I still be struggling to walk now? Would the walk to work still be one of my greatest fears and yet one of my biggest goals? If I had done everything wrong would my cards have been dealt in the same unfortunate way? All questions I suppose like 'Who came first, the chicken or the egg?' All questions that nobody will ever have the answer to.

Will Stephanie Millward ever know the cause of her MS?

Will she ever have the cure? No, probably not. Her cards obviously haven't been dealt that way.

CHAPTER 3
Jeddah, Saudi Arabia

My life began in Baskh hospital, Jeddah, Saudi Arabia. Weighing 7.1 pounds I was almost half a pound lighter than my older brother, Paul, and then the same difference between my younger sister Kristy and younger brother Nicholas who were all 7 pounds and 6 ounces. I suppose I was the odd one out even then!

Jeddah conjours up wonderful feelings and memories of being loved and happy; all but for one instance when I vividly remember going to the local surgery for an inoculation. I hid underneath the doctor's couch to try to stay away from the great big terrifying needle but eventually I was dragged out by the doctor and my mum. This was when my fear of needles first started and this fear still remains with me now even after having to learn how to inject myself at the tender age of eighteen. I often think that even the darkest fears are summoned for us to face and get over, as though perhaps we are not allowed to be scared of anything. I was incredibly thankful that I had my BCG injection when I was born and I therefore didn't have to see the needle and I don't have to bear the ugly scar that most teenagers have to endure for life.

The sun shone constantly in Saudi Arabia and because of my happy memories there I associate the sun with me being happy. It was something that I could always rely on. The memories of such a fantastic and luxurious place fill my mind with a sense of fun and of pure elation. These wonderful feelings and memories always make me smile. I was leading such a fantastic life having being born in Jeddah; I wouldn't have swapped lives with anyone.

The sun created a temperature of approximately 40 degrees every day and in the summer that rose to almost unbearable temperatures of around 55 degrees. We had to wear sun cream all the time and stay in the shade where possible but the all year tan and almost white, shiny blonde hair were an attractive consequence! I feel that the summer's extra heat was just another excuse to go on holiday, which we did every year.

As a family we often travelled to exotic locations such as Bangkok, Greece, Italy and Athens when it was too hot for us in Saudi Arabia. While in Bangkok we often saw elephant shows and visited rose gardens and other attractions. Watching an elephant show one time I remember two elephants putting their trunks together, then my mum sat on their trunks and she was raised up in the air where we took a picture of her terrified face! We also went to camel parades where the camels bent down to the ground so that we could climb on their backs before they stood up. I am surprised none of us fell off! My little brother, Nicholas, liked snakes so one day we went to a snake show and a cobra was put around his neck. I was scared for him as Nicholas was my best friend. We always stayed together all day long. Be careful, be nice; he won't hurt you then. Nicholas loved it all!

There was a pool approximately fifty metres away from where we lived and my parents tried to teach us to swim from an early age. While I was still in nappies I walked to the edge of the pool, fell in and swam like a mermaid - or rather, like a rock - and sank to the bottom before my brother, Paul, shouted for my dad to 'Get Stephanie out before she drowns!'

Obviously, after this experience I was terrified of water and even having a shower or washing my face was difficult and ended with me in a complete stress and a puddle of tears. My mum and dad worked very hard to get me to have a shower quietly. Then, when I started getting more confident with water, I was reintroduced to the pool. I apparently just got in and swam like a fish.

My parents enrolled us into a swimming club called Saudi Sharks and we trained there often during the week and went to competitions at the weekend. Some of the competitions were just inter-club championships where you fought for your place on the squad; others were national championships against people from all over Saudi Arabia. I did well in these championships and was invited to swim in Riyadh (the capital of Saudi Arabia) to compete in the Junior Olympics aged eight. I won this event as I did many more!

I had a friend in Saudi who lived in the house behind mine. He was one of my best friends and we played together all day. Richard did everything with and for me. I made him come round to my house for dinner and I remember having a problem cooking baked beans. We both now hate the taste and the texture just because of this one meal we had at my house. Sorry, Richard! I remember making Richard do ballet dancing practices with me. He was not the most able ballet dancer but his devotion to our friendship made him try all the time, uncomplaining. A true friend.

When Nicholas was born, in 1985, he then became my best friend, following me around everywhere. We did everything together and I played with him and his toys which we both loved. Nicholas had the cutest face so even when he did something wrong you couldn't tell him off. It was nice having two brothers and one sister, and the four of us made up a very strong team with my mum and dad leading us.

Leigh, Manchester, United Kingdom; the home of my grandparents

Every time we visited my grandparents it rained, and almost all the time over the periods we were staying in the UK it rained. Rain caused everyone to stay inside and complain about the weather! I remember asking my mum why it rained and she said it was to feed the trees and the flowers. This seemed like a good reason for rain but it seemed to rain a lot for the number of trees and other plants there were! Maybe it rains so much in one country because in deserts, like Saudi Arabia, it barely ever rains. I do remember the only time in the ten years I lived in Jeddah when it did rain. It was like a celebration and all my friends and I went out on our bikes riding around and enjoying the refreshing feel of water as opposed to sun on our skin. We all enjoyed this new experience and it was a shame when the sun came back and was twice as strong as it had been originally.

School, Jeddah

I travelled to my school, on a bus every day which was an exciting experience because it was a large school and therefore had a number of buses coming to the school grounds. I always met my friend, Mandy, when I got off the bus. Mandy had only one leg so she came into the school by taxi and she always had her crutches which were incredibly fun to play with. If Mandy needed to go to the toilet while she was at school one person had to go with her to the nurse and the nurse would help Mandy go to the toilet. Whenever I got chosen to take Mandy to the nurse I felt very proud and important. I loved helping Mandy.

I also had many friends from different countries and from different religions. One of my friends was a Muslim so during Ramadan she couldn't eat in the daylight as it was against her religion. Another friend was from Canada originally, so she told me all about Canada and of the things she did in the summer breaks.

Everybody's experiences were very exciting and intriguing and I feel privileged to have met so many people from different backgrounds as I feel it has made me a better person. I remember going to the town centre with my mum and dad and all the locals loved my blonde hair and white skin. They grabbed our faces and shook them for what seemed like hours in a sort of amazed but caressing way. Kristy and I laughed about it afterwards as it seemed like such a strange thing to do!

On a school trip once, I was taken to the desert to camp outside so that we could experience the different temperatures. During the day it was incredibly hot but at night the temperatures were the other extreme and it was very cold. My dad was asked to help the teachers so he was allowed to come on the trip too! During the day we went around the desert looking at the plants that lived there and we saw some of the animals and insects that live in the desert. Then, in the evening, we sat around a bonfire singing loads of songs and eating hamburgers and hot dogs. This was very enjoyable until my dad noticed a large scorpion who wanted to join in the fun. It was quite scary as we had been told all about scorpions and how poisonous they are. My dad moved the scorpion away from the bonfire. I was very proud of my dad; he was so brave!

At the age of nine and a half the Gulf war forced my family to give up its easy tax-free life in exchange for Great Britain where people had strange accents and only had occasional holidays. I was used to going to gorgeous places like Bangkok a couple of times a year as well as travelling from Jeddah to stay with my grandparents in Leigh, England for the main holidays such as Christmas, Easter and for the summer holiday. My grandparents' accents had always interested me as with our American accents my family sounded very posh in comparison to everyone else! People still ask me about my strange twang which apparently can be anything from South African to Australian!

Bilbo

My grandparents owned a Shetland pony called Bilbo who used to be a gymkhana pony but who always seemed to be very bad tempered and hated being ridden or touched. If he got the chance he would take a huge chunk out of your arm! Bilbo was very vicious but we still insisted on riding him. These riding experiences always ended the same way with each of us galloping around the field holding on for dear life and then finally being bucked off and landing in the middle of the field crying while the pony sweetly picking at some sweet grass nearby. We never learned and every time we were back in Manchester we would give Bilbo another chance! One of my relatives had a large livery yard with normal horses which would have been a safer option than trying to stay on Bilbo's back. My cousin, Kate, is about three months older than me and we got on very well so I often went to the farm to help out with mucking out the stables and riding the horses. Once, while I was there, we were feeding the horses and Kate's horse,

Carlos, decided to bang on the stable door continuously until Kate gave him some lager in his food. An alcoholic horse!

I loved these trips to the farm especially when, on one occasion, Kate had found a horse called Gemma which she said would be perfect to buy. I rode Gemma round the field in front of my dad and led her over a few jumps. She was a wonderful horse and did everything I asked her to do. My dad decided that we were not going to buy Gemma because we had nowhere to keep her and because I would have to spend too much time looking after her and would not concentrate on my school work or my swimming. I was annoyed that I couldn't have my own horse but I knew that it was probably better to concentrate on school.

Every year for Easter my grandparents bought us a huge box of Mini Eggs. These never lasted very long but they were a wonderful present! My grandparents always had a number of dogs in their house so we had a lot of fun throwing the eggs for the dogs to catch as well as eating our own handfuls! During my early years, I decided that I wanted lots of dogs, lots of horses and lots of Mini Eggs when I grew up. I had counted on winning the Olympic Games and meeting a very rich guy to marry; possibly Sean Connery or at least a look-a-like! Everything seemed so easy. It was all going to work out as planned.

The dreams of a child, so fresh and so happy. It is a shame they all had to change for me.

CHAPTER 4

Wiltshire's Junior Swimmer of the Year, 1998

From the age of twelve to fifteen I was swimming for Corsham Amateur Swimming Club ASC with coaches Peggy Tanner and Julia Airlie, and I loved every minute of it: I loved the training, I loved the hard work and I loved knowing I was good at something! Paul, Kristy and Nicholas also swam for Corsham and we enjoyed the competitions that we went to. Actually, maybe Nicholas didn't like swimming as much as I did but he did enjoy screaming for us when we were racing and he did enjoy reading his books when no one was racing. Paul loved the competitions and the desire to win, to push himself as far as he could go. Kristy just liked the chatting in between sets and on the poolside before and after and she loved getting changed where she didn't stop talking.

At Corsham there were other good swimmers that we raced against in training and who we enjoyed competing with: Sara and Matt Croften, David Lawrence and Rebecca McCrae were especially good.

The presentation evening for our club championships was one of the highlights of the year. We all went out bought new outfits, new shoes and had a hair cut ready for the evening. Kristy and I spent hours getting ready with my mum, who also enjoyed helping.

Mum often curled our hair into soft curls; my soft curls fell out almost straight away even with the many gallons of hairspray on it. My hair is very straight and it likes being straight. It doesn't believe in soft curls and therefore remains straight. Kristy's hair was a lot more versatile and her soft curls stayed in longer allowing Kristy to look stunning all night!

Driving to the local community centre was always an exciting time. We knew we were going to have a great night and that we were going to be bringing back loads of medals and cups home! Every presentation evening was a success and it offered motivation for the whole year. I think my dad loved being in charge of carrying boxes full of medals back to the car! I wish to thank everyone involved in these affairs as they were truly marvellous.

I received an invitation to the West of England's Sports Personality of the Year in 1998 and I was excited and surprised about this invitation. Have I won? Just imagine if I have! Wow! I went to the evening dressed up in a new outfit specially bought for this special evening. It reminded me of the presentation evenings with Corsham ASC. I don't normally drink fizzy drinks but at the presentation evenings and at this swimmer of the year event I allowed myself to have a glass of Coke which was exciting in itself. My parents had come to the evening too and we sat at a table with our drinks waiting for the introductions. Both my mum and I were people-watching to see if we recognised anyone famous. I found this evening very exciting and when the nominations for the Junior Sports Person of the Year were called out I could feel the nerves in my stomach. In the end I did win and was awarded Wiltshire's Junior Swimmer of the year, 1998. I was also given £200 which was supposed to be used for sports equipment to help make me stronger and therefore help with my training. I bought a treadmill which I loved using. Kristy and I had made it a regime to go for a run just about every day but this was definitely easier! I was thrilled with my award and loved the evening. I couldn't wait to win some more awards and to hopefully get to the Olympic Games. Wiltshire's Junior Sports Personality of the year! Wow, what a prize!

My mum asked Bath University if I could train up there with the other swimmers as I was swimming very well with Corsham ASC but I needed more pool time to enable me to get faster and stronger. I was allowed to go on a trial and was accepted to train with David Lyles as my coach! David was a kind man who started originally coaching Swindon's Tigersharks swimming team before moving around the country to other venues. Eventually, David was asked to be the head coach of the Chinese team in Shanghai and then the New Zealand team! For me, David became a friend who helped me perfect my swimming technique and he helped with my motivation!

Sydney Olympic Games, 2000, here I come!

CHAPTER 5

Swimming for Bath University, 1995-99

Beeeeeep! The sound of the alarm clock woke me and as per usual I rushed to wake up before struggling to get into my costume then throwing my school uniform and shoes on. Pulling my hair into a ponytail with an elastic band I moved in front of the mirror to I brushed my teeth. I felt excited about the sessions for today. I had been working very hard up until this week because the National Championships were getting closer so I needed to start tapering. I had been doing some quick split times in training so I hoped to swim a good time at the National Championships.

My dad came into my room pushing me to get out the door.

'Are you ready?' he asked.

'Just need to grab some lunch,' I replied.

Rushing out the door I saw the clock: 05.15. Late again. Maybe I should have left my lunch?

We jump in my dad's car and start driving onto the A4. I am sure my dad drove a little too fast but as there were no other cars on the road there was no one around to complain. It took us about twenty minutes to get to Bath University, park the car then run inside to the sports centre. The clock showed 05.40. Yes! I made it!

I ran onto the poolside where Andy Clayton, Jaime King and a few other swimmers were already stretching. David Lyles and Ian Turner, the coaches, were in their office. I started my normal stretches to loosen up.

The clock struck 06.00 and we all moved to the end of the pool ready to dive in. Lane 2 is my lane and as I normally led it, I stood on the top of the starting block. Knowing that the pool would be freezing cold, apparently the proper swimming temperature, I shivered excitedly.

'Swimmers, are you ready?' David's loud voice made me jump. 'Go!'

I was in the pool and didn't notice the temperature change until I started swimming freestyle. It was absolutely freezing and I was already desperate to get out and I hadn't even finished the first 50m! I tried to swim a little faster to get a bit warmer. The wall was nearing. Yes, I said to myself. The initial shock was over and I was ready to concentrate on my swimming. The warm-up consisted of 800m freestyle with every fourth length backstroke. I felt very strong and enjoyed the session. The total distance for the session was 6200m. I stretched again then went to the changing rooms for a quick shower. I had to rush because my dad still had to get to Swindon to start his job and I had to get to Corsham for school. I was allowed to be late for registration every day but was not allowed to be late for first lesson which started at 08:40.

Running out of the sports centre I saw my dad in his car. I ran as fast as I could before coming to a dead halt and swinging the door open, pushing myself inside, my swimming bag still on my back. My dad drove me to school where he kissed me on the cheek and I ran into one of the school blocks. I pulled my bag around to the front and opened the folder to see which class I was supposed to be in. Physics, oh no! The science rooms were at the other end of the school. I ran the three hundred metres then dashed up the stairs to my physics room. Knocking on the door I remembered that I hadn't done my homework. I went into the room and found a place next to Laura. She smiled at me.

'Welcome, Stephanie,' said my teacher.

I smiled in return.

It was very warm in this class. Maybe it was the panting I was doing after that run!

I enjoyed physics so the hour lesson went by very quickly and I went on to maths where we had an algebra test for ten minutes; no calculators allowed. I have always been good at maths so the test was quite easy, thankfully. We then went on to completing a past paper on simultaneous equations.

There was a twenty minute break after the maths lesson so I ate my breakfast before going to my Spanish lesson. When I got to class, the Spanish teacher started chatting away to me in Spanish but I was lost after the first word so was uncertain how to reply. 'Umm...' I decided to say 'I live in a house' as this might have been the right answer.

'What type of house?' he asked in Spanish.

Yes! I had chosen the right answer. 'A bungalow,' I replied with a smile on my face. He went on to ask Brett where he lived and what kind of house it was. I must be such a lucky person to have got that question right!

Spanish finished and was followed by English where we were dissecting the novel 'Frankenstein'. As homework I needed to write an essay about chapter ten of this book.

English finished: 13.00, lunch time. I went over to where the head teacher and my mother had their offices. My mum worked as the head teacher's secretary. Seeing my mum through the window I smiled and she smiled back. I sat in the reception and ate my sandwich before my mum walked out.

'Are you OK?' she asked.

'Yeah, I'm great!' I replied.

I followed her to her car and we climbed in. My mum started the car and she drove me back to Bath University before driving back to the school to finish her work at 16.00. Today was a Wednesday and every Wednesday I was allowed to go to the university for the last hour of school as it was a PE lesson. At the university I went for a three mile run around the University campus and then went into the fitness room to do a beast of an abs session including thousands of sit-ups and press-ups. The circuit training was always hard work and then we were back in the pool at 16.00 for another two hour session.

18.00 arrived and my mum was sitting in the seating arena waiting to take me home. I was very excited as I had worked hard today! We got home at 18.40 and my mum heated my dinner in the oven for me. She had cooked dinner when she had finished work and Kristy, Paul and Nicholas had already eaten theirs but mine was obviously cold by now. I finished my meal then went to my room to write that English essay about 'Frankenstein'.

With the essay complete I collected a dry towel and packed it into my swimming bag ready for the next morning then I fell asleep at 22:30 ready for Thursday. The same alarm woke me the next morning and the same routine was followed. Wednesdays were the hard days where we had to do the land work as well as the swimming. On the other week days we had to swim 06.00 to 08.00 then 16.00 to 18.00. The weekends were easy as there were no sessions on Saturday and only one session on Sunday. We were also allowed one session off during the week which was generally a Tuesday or a Thursday morning.

I really enjoyed everything about training at Bath University and I was very much looking forward to my first major competition swimming for them. This competition was going to be the National Age Group Championships to be held in Coventry. A year ago I had swum the 100m Butterfly in this competition in Crystal Palace and had come twentieth, even after spending a fortnight on a water sports holiday with my school just before racing! This year I intended to do a number of events from the 200m Butterfly to 100m Backstroke. I was very excited about this competition as after all the training I was hoping for some fast times! I started training at Bath University aged just fourteen but my life was about to hit an ultimate immense peak before then sinking into a dark and treacherous trough signalling the end to my perfect existence.

CHAPTER 6

National Age Group
Championships, 1997

'Wally, you looked so good in the warm-up. Are you looking forward to the race?' My best friend Amy Howland had a huge smile on her face.

'Yeah, I felt very good,' I replied. Amy and I had been best friends for a long time and we called each other Wally and Wazzy.

We were both in the changing rooms at the pool in Coventry. I was changing from my warm-up costume to my white racing costume. My white costume was a wonderful invention! Every time I wore this costume I won the race! I have never lost or even come second with the white costume on! I only wore the white costume when I swam backstroke races just in case it didn't work as well for the butterfly races!

I was due to swim in heat four of the eight heats for the 100m Backstroke and I was allocated lane 6. I was looking forward to this race as I was anticipating a good time after all the training at Bath Uni.

'Stephanie, they are calling for your event now.' My mum looked excited about my swim.

'Cool!' I replied and started walking to the call-up room.

'Good luck,' my mum replied.

'Thank you!'

Amy and my mum moved into the seating area where they were going to cheer for me. My dad, Kristy, Paul, Nicholas and Sylvia (Amy's mum) were already seated and chatting excitedly to each other. I walked over to my coach, David Lyles, who was stood on the poolside waiting for me.

'How are you feeling?' he asked.

'Yeah, very good,' I replied. I couldn't wait to get in the pool, truthfully, just to see how good I was.

'Go out hard, do a fast turn then come back strong. Work the underwater parts. See how far you can go,' David instructed on how to swim the race.

Julia Airlie was standing close by. 'Just enjoy it,' she added. Julia was one of the coaches at Corsham ASC and she was a good friend. She always knew how to correct a stroke technique and she was a sweet person.

'Fast start and fast turn,' Peggy said. Peggy was the head coach at Corsham ASC.

It was wonderful that the whole team had come to cheer me on!

'Lane 6 Stephanie Millward.' One of the helpers was getting the swimmers in line ready for the heats.

'Yes,' I called, stepping forward. I was stood in line for my heat.

'Good luck,' David said before taking his place with the other coaches on the poolside.

I turned around and looked at the pool. Just two lengths of this 50m pool and then I'd know how fast I was! I was mentally prepared for the swim when heat six was called up to stand behind the starting blocks.

The whistle blew for silence in the pool area.

'Go Stephanie!' I heard Nicholas call.

Smiling, I put my right arm up to receive the remark.

The whistle instructed us to get in the pool ready for the start.

'Swimmers, take your marks.' Pulling forward and hunching myself up taut against the wall I was ready to do my backstroke start.

The gun shot sounded and my body flew into action. My arms

were spinning round and round. 'Keep your head still' I remembered Peggy saying. I could hear the cheering in the pool and I could imagine everyone shouting for me.

'Go Stephanie,' I told myself.

The five metre flags were above me which meant I had three strokes my turn. The five metre flags are used as an indicator of where the wall is and help swimmers prepare to either turn or finish. The turn was OK for me but I was a little too far away from the wall so the push off wasn't very powerful. I'll have to swim harder, I was thinking, to counteract the push off the wall. Work the arms, I was telling myself. Go faster. The five metre flags were above me again. Yes! I had almost finished, just the five metres into the wall.

My right hand hit the wall hard and I turned to see the time: 1 minute 6 seconds 56! Wow, I thought, what a wonderful time! I had swum faster than ever before which was fantastic. I had won the heat by quite a long way too and I had to wait until everyone had finished racing before I could get out.

'Well done!' I heard my family call. I smiled up at them. I had just knocked about ten seconds off my original personal best time. I was amazed and very excited!

'You are in the final, Stephanie,' David said after my swim-down when I went to see him for a review of my race. 'Lane 4 first place into the final.'

Wow! The fastest swimmer into the final! I was awarded lane four which would allow me to see all my competitors as it is one of the two centre lanes!

First place! Wow! First place so far, anyway. The Olympic dream beckoned. I might get to go to the Olympics after all.

I spent lunch time running through my swim with my coach and then finding a big jacket potato to eat. Coming back into the changing rooms with my mum we heard two girls talking in one of the changing cubicles.

'Where did she come from? Stephanie wasn't even at the Nationals last year.'

'I don't know. She looked very good.'

Both my mum and I smiled. They obviously didn't know we were listening to their conversation!

I swam my warm-up for the final feeling very confident and very excited. 'Mum I'm going to win this race', I said with a smile on my face.

'Don't say that. Someone might knock lots of time off and beat you.'

'No,' I replied. 'I'm going to win'. And that is exactly what I did, with a new British age group record time of 1.05.68. Just think, last year I hadn't even qualified for a place in the heats of the 100m Backstroke and this year I won the whole event! I was over the moon with the result.

Next, I swam the 200m Backstroke in the time of 2.22.34 coming third, the 200m Butterfly in 2.20 and came fifth and the 100m Butterfly in 1.08 and came seventh. Fifteen years old and I was the best in the country. Fifteen years old with all my dreams in my hands!

After these wonderful performances I went back to training with an added passion and worked extra hard! My story was in the local papers with headlines implying an Olympic champion. The dreams were coming alive and I was as high as a kite! My life was perfect and I was loving every single minute of it. One day I would be an Olympic champion with many Olympic medals! This was my goal and it was working out perfectly! An Olympic gold medal was the dream and the passion and my life story was playing one hundred percent correctly.

Stephanie Millward, Olympic Champion, is just round the corner!

CHAPTER 7

Swimming for Great Britain Senior Team, 1998

After the excitement of the Nationals had died down a little I came home from swimming one day to find another important letter waiting for me. I opened the envelope, read the letter and then went running round the house showing everyone!

'I have been asked to swim in two World Cup events for Great Britain Senior Team!'

I was only fifteen years old and one of the best swimmers in the country which is why I was chosen for this event. WOW! My dreams were alive!

'Mum! I am being taken to Sweden and Germany to swim for the Great Britain senior team! Dad, Paul, Kristy, Nicholas, everybody! I am going to swim for Great Britain!' I couldn't come to terms with the fact that I was going to represent my country! I took my letter into school the next day and showed everybody. They were all very proud and very excited for me and my teachers were amazed at my success, but then my mum noticed something very important.

'Stephanie, your swimming trip is when you will be doing your GCSE exams. Your geography exam.'

What? I had to swim for England now that I had been asked. It was the chance of a lifetime.

'Maybe you can do the exam while you are over in Sweden?

Maybe I thought, maybe.

It was agreed that I could do my geography GCSE exam while I was in Sweden. I had to swim my 100m Backstroke heats in the morning, come back to the hotel for my exam and then go back to the pool for the finals. That can't be too hard, I thought.

My exams started while I was in hard training and very tired so without any revision I took my exams. They seemed to be going well so when I started to taper again and had more energy I started looking through some of my books ready for my geography exam.

Flying out to Malmo, Sweden, as part of the GB team, I felt very proud and excited. We were all dressed in our team kit and attracted a lot of attention. I was swimming for my country along with all these other excellent Olympic swimmers and it made me feel so good and so incredibly proud!

We arrived in Sweden where we rode in a minibus to take us to our five star hotel. I was given a room to share with another swimmer, which was nice as I made a friend. Dinner was a delicious experience because the whole team was there at the same time and the swimmers ate loads which meant that the assistants had to keep ordering more food!

The pool in Malmo was full of salt water which tasted awful; every time I swam I had to make a conscious effort not to swallow any of the water. It seemed strange to be swimming in a pool with salt water being used to fight infections in the water as opposed to chlorine. I was thankful to get out of the salt water and to have a fresh water shower!

The day when I was due to swim the 100m Backstroke came and I was a little worried and a little nervous. I never normally felt nervous so this was a strange feeling for me. I lined up for the race as I had done many times before. I smiled, realising I had gone to places people have only ever dreamed of. I was here, in Sweden, swimming for Great Britain! I was one of the best swimmers in the whole world! I swam a good race in a time of 1.06.54. This was fast enough for me to qualify for the final.

After my swim-down I had to rush with one of the coaches back to the hotel. Here I was instructed to sit in a room for three hours answering the Geography questions. I had just reached the finals so I didn't really want to be doing this exam. I was now an international swimmer: what did I need school for now? I will be offered lots of money and sponsorship deals to swim, I don't need good grades! All these thoughts flew through my mind as I wrote.

I rushed through the exam anxious to get back to the pool and ready for my final. The swimming coach told me to pick up some lunch so we sat in the cafeteria before leaving the hotel. I was getting scared that I would miss my race. We got back in plenty of time for me to have another warm-up before putting on my Great Britain racing costume. It had the GB flag on it and it made me feel very special.

'Stephanie, how did your GCSE exam go?' I felt so young and that everyone was laughing at me. What was I doing going for an exam while I was swimming for Great Britain?

'Yeah, it was OK!' I answered with a quick smile.

My final was good and I swam very strongly. I finished in seventh place in a similar time to the heats 1.06.45 which meant that I was seventh in the world! This meant that I was definitely going to the Sydney Olympics in 2000! I was fast enough. I am going to go to the Olympics. I am very good and I will succeed as an international swimmer. After school this will be my job. I will get paid just to swim! What a wonderful life. How exciting!

When the trials in Sweden were complete we flew out direct to Gelsenkirchen, Germany. In Germany we were to swim the same events but against a slightly different selection of competitors. We were taken to stay in another fantastic five star hotel! Therewere some well-known fast swimmers and while travelling up for lunch I got into the same lift as Alexander Popov! I fell in love at first sight; he was stunning! I was in a two metre squared lift with a man I loved! Looking back I should have opened my mouth and spoken to him but I was so excited that I was in the lift, just me and him, and I was speechless! I went home with a smile plastered on my face.

Arriving home my mum questioned how much I enjoyed the trip

and I answered, 'I have met the man I want to marry – Alexander Popov! He is so nice and handsome!'

'I am not sure that is very practical,' my mum answered.

Oh well, I thought, I can keep dreaming!

That year I went to the British Championships (Nationals) and won a gold medal in the 100m Backstroke swimming a 1.05.16, and two silvers for the 50m and the 200m Backstroke. I felt absolutely wonderful. I was a good swimmer, the best in the whole country, and I was going to win the Olympics. Everything was wonderful and my life was excellent. I was living my dream!

CHAPTER 8

World Schools Games, 1998

Following the successful World Cup events I was invited to swim for Great Britain in the World Schools Championships in Shanghai, China in 1998. I was chosen to swim the 100m Backstroke, 200m Backstroke and the 100m Backstroke in the team relay.

I was swimming so very well that I was bound to do well in China. I had never been there before so I was very excited for that reason too. Recently, I had moved up to swim with Ian Turner where I trained with amazing swimmers like Paul Palmer and Andy Clayton! These sessions were harder as they were further and faster; I really must be a proper Olympic possibility now!

Two weeks before we were booked to fly to China I got a cold and bad earache which really annoyed me. I never get sick. Why did I have to get sick now? I also had to go for a hepatitis A injection which would apparently stop me from getting hepatitis A which can be transported in water.

I went to the doctors with my mum to get my injection, both of us thinking and feeling that this was a bad idea because I wasn't rid of the earache yet. The injection could prevent an illness but for me it could have caused one. We asked the doctor whether I was allowed to have the injection as I was ill already with the cold. Yes, he said even though I still had a temperature. I had the injection and straight away I had an awful feeling that I had done the wrong thing. This was to be a life-changing decision that would be the end of everything I loved and indeed an awful decision with reactions that were endless and all very bad for me.

I still went to China feeling not very well and knowing somehow that this time I was not going to get better. While in China I came eighth in both of my individual races and second in the relay. I should have won all my races as I was seeded first but I felt awful from the cold and earache and swam some bad times. The nightmare had begun.

I met some very nice swimmers while on this camp and on one day after the swimming was over and we were enjoying the gymnastics, someone had the bright idea that we should try to stay up all night and just drink lots of alcohol! We all agreed that this was a wonderful idea and so started straight away. The shops seemed to have very cheap drinks which just encouraged s to buy more and more. We had a great time drinking and chatting and we stayed up all or at least the majority of the night. The next night we did very much the same thing even though we were feeling pretty tired. On the last night, even though we were shattered, we had to try to keep our eyes open and when we got on the coach to drive back to the airport, our eyes drooped and often closed. We remained excited that we had stayed awake for three nights but the trip home was very hard and we all fell asleep on our bags in the airport while waiting for the plane. It was a nice end to my life as a Great Britain Olympic swimmer (almost) and it will remain in my mind forever.

I went home feeling nauseous and unsteady as well as shattered from the lack of sleep. My mum said the colour had gone from my face and she told me to go straight to bed. The next day I seemed to be getting worse and so my mum booked an appointment to see the doctor. The doctor was unsure why I was feeling so bad and said I should see an ENT (Ear, Nose and Throat) doctor. My mum booked for me in for a private appointment which cost my parents five hundred pounds.

The ENT doctor noticed an unusual flutter in the pupils in my eyes and advised me to see a neurologist because the problem definitely was not in my ears, nose or throat. Coincidently there was a neurologist standing outside of the room. He came in, did a few tests and told me to go for an MRI (Magnetic Resonance Imaging - a brain scan) and to see him the next day for results. I was terrified. What was wrong with my brain? Did I have a brain tumour?

Hopefully this will all be nothing and I will be given a course of antibiotics and everything will be fine. What would I do if he says I am going to die? Is this why I swam so badly in China? Have I just got a cold? It doesn't feel like just a cold maybe it is glandular fever or the flu? I don't want to die, I am too young. I haven't been to the Olympics yet. The worrying thoughts raced through my mind.

I feel it is somehow appropriate that my swimming career ended in China in 1998. I couldn't have known then that swimming would bring me back to China again on another bitter-sweet occasion later in life. China and its pitiful experiences will with me forever so I chose to have a tattoo, the Chinese symbol for LOVE imprinted on the back of my shoulder. The tattoo is forever and I needed to keep my true love alive forever too.

My life then turned very hard and dark and the love I have for my family and close friends is the only reason I am still alive now. I hit the deepest, darkest part of any hole and hopefully nobody else ever gets this low. If you have a bad feeling about something, please listen to your body or your mind. It might save your life.

CHAPTER 9

The Brain Scan, 7th May 1999

Arriving at the hospital I felt very nervous and worried. A brain scan? Only very sick people have a brain scan and this is normally when they have a brain tumour or some other brain illness. I only have an infection; I don't need a brain scan. Walking up to the hospital I walked into the bush by the side of the path three times. I felt very silly; why was I doing such a strange thing? Nobody walks into the bush unless they are drunk! Opening the door I felt a cold gust of air. The white walls looked so angry and the putrid smell of disinfectant covered the whole of my face. I had a nauseating feeling and I could smell death.

I felt nervous when I met the nurse who was going to do my scan. She was dressed all in white – clean. She seemed too happy, too correct. Is she looking at me as a very sick person who has to have her brain checked just in case? What a strange and terrifying feeling. I didn't want the scan in case it told me the wrong thing. If it told me I was going to die what would I do? I gave my mum a smile to give her some confidence. Cover the pain, hide the truth.

I lay flat on my back with my head strapped down to keep it motionless. The buzzing sound numbed my mind and made me think about all the bad possibilities. If something was really wrong what would I do? Lots of people unexpectedly get sick and die. Will I be one of them? I haven't done enough with my life yet. I want to go to the Olympics.

'Stay still; it is almost done,' said the nurse.

Was I really going to move anywhere with all this strapping?

'OK, that scan is finished. I will start the second one in a few moments.'

How many of these scans am I going to have? Are the scans killing my brain cells? Are they wiping out the rest of my short-term memories?

The buzzing started again and I tried to be motionless, even holding my breath. It seemed to take forever before finally the buzzing stopped. The nurse again said that there would be a couple of minutes before she started the next scan.

I must be dying. Nobody has all these scans for no reason. There must be a huge tumour sitting in my brain and the nurse is just seeing how long it will be before I stop breathing. This thought was terrifying. Just imagine if my fears were true. I haven't said goodbye yet.

After six scans the nurse said that she had finished and she started to undo all of the locks that were holding me down.

'Am I going to die' I asked her, hoping for a good answer.

'No, but I am not qualified to tell you what is wrong. I am only qualified to take the scan.'

OK, so she can't tell me about the tumour on the brain. I had an appointment the next day with the neurologist so he would be able to tell me what was wrong. This evening will feel like waiting for Christmas, just without the presents the next day. What's going to happen? Am I really sick? Am I going to die tonight in bed? Obviously I was very worried when I went to bed and so I opened the door letting Spring follow me into bed. Spring offered me the comfort I so desperately needed. If I die at least I will die a happy person.

CHAPTER 10

Results, 8th May 1999 and 24th September 1999

8th May 1999 – Last day at Bath University as a swimmer

I went to Bath as usual today for my swimming session and felt fine but just a little worried about the results of the MRI scan which was where I was going after the swimming session. Everything was going in exactly the same way as usual until I was told to swim a set of 100m freestyles off the turn-around time of one minute and thirty seconds. I started OK but then I couldn't quite see the clock's hands and I couldn't therefore make out the times I was supposed to be swimming off. I struggled with my poor eyesight thinking that it was just a momentary thing and that I would be fine, but then I swam straight into the wall instead of turning in front of it. This seemed very strange, and so when I swam into another swimmer I felt it only right to get out of the pool for a break before I caused some damage.

Ian Turner, my amazing coach, said that it was fine to get out and his then-wife, Kerrie, was on the poolside. I put both hands on the poolside as usual to get out but slipped right back in again; my arms had no strength. Try again. This time I fell flat on the poolside with two of the swimmers helping to push me out and Ian and his wife pulling me out. I felt stupid and apologised profusely. Ian then told me to go home and rest and only come back when I was well.

That day turned out to be my last training at Bath University with Ian Turner and David Lyles. A pain-filled memory and a day I will never forget.

After having a shower and getting changed I went over to my mum and dad. I could see the fear in their eyes and as soon as my mum smiled I burst out crying.

'What's wrong with me?'

I remember Mum putting her arms around me and hugging me hard as I tried to control the tears. I have to be strong for everyone as well as for myself.

'We have to see the scan and hear the results. We need to be as strong as possible just in case,' she replied, comforting me,

My dad drove the three of us to the hospital where we were having the meeting with the neurologist, Dr Kenneth Dawson. I had nerves in my stomach but I decided to ignore them and spoke about easy subjects asking, for example, what we were having for dinner that night.

Getting to the hospital I climbed out of the car. Remembering my last trip to the hospital when I walked into the bush by the path three times I studied the path and I fully concentrated on where I was placing my feet. I got to the hospital without the burden of having hit the bush! The lift took us up and we walked out, each of us looking at the door of the neurologist's room with dread. What was he going to tell us?

The neurologist asked me how I felt and I said fine. He then went on to say he had been looking at my scan results and it showed a lot of swelling and scarring on my brain. Scars? I am only seventeen years old, why would I have scars on my brain?

'Your illness could be an infection; Lupus or Multiple Sclerosis. We will have to wait a bit longer to find out which one it is.'

What? I was hoping it was an infection.

The neurologist went on to ask what we had thought it was. I said I thought it was just an infection. My mum thought it was a brain tumour and my dad thought I had Mad Cow's disease – thanks dad!

At least I didn't have a tumour as I had feared. At least I wasn't going to die just yet. The neurologist kept saying that it could be just an infection but I could tell he knew otherwise but just wasn't telling us yet. It could be Lupus or MS. Which would be better? I hadn't heard of either before so hopefully they were not too bad. When the neurologist told me to stand outside while he had a quick conversation with my mum and dad I felt terrified. Maybe I am going to die and he is telling my parents how bad I am or maybe he is saying about all the pain I am going to be in or maybe he is saying that my life is over. When I was allowed back in I saw the fear in my parents' eyes. Great, bad news, obviously.

I was shown pictures from the scan which showed the many scars on my brain. It seemed strange that the photo was an image of what was inside my head and that something was attacking me, making me sick. If I stay positive and happy no one will see my fears. If I stay the same as normal maybe the illness will get better. I shouldn't be sick, I never get sick. Maybe the scan showed someone else's brain and mine was fine. I don't believe that I have got a disease in my brain, not at seventeen and definitely not when I am meant to be going to the Sydney Olympic Games next year. Maybe this is all just a very bad dream.

Going home I was happy and positive, it was obviously just a bad infection, I will be back soon. A bad infection unfortunately that will never go away. The neurologist had told my parents that he was worried about the amount of scarring on my brain and that he thought it was MS, an incurable illness of the central nervous system. He told me nothing and I kept the usual positive persona alive: the depression was just round the corner but I still had the dreams and the high goals - the Olympic Games, the medals yet to be won. I was still happy, living life to the full, enjoying every day with all its amazing events. I was living the dream and loving every moment. Today was just a blip in the program, nothing was wrong really. Everything will be fine tomorrow.

Unfortunately for me that tomorrow never came. Six months later I received the confirmation of my illness.

CHAPTER 11

What is Multiple Sclerosis? (It never needs to be the end)

MS is an autoimmune disease. This means that the immune system of an MS sufferer attacks their own body. In the case of an MS patient, the central nervous system (the brain and the spinal cord) is the affected area of the body. As yet, there is no known reason behind why the immune system attacks the body's own cells. I try to treat MS as me in a bad mood and I therefore have to stay in a good or at least positive mood! Basically whenever I am angry, sad, tired or frustrated the MS gets more powerful and attacks me. My bad days are caused by negative energy so therefore I need to stay positive to keep a control of the illness.

The myelin sheath

The main thing that is happening in MS is that the body's own immune system is attacking the myelin sheath that surrounds our nerve cells. Myelin surrounds and insulates the nerve fibres and allows the transfer of messages from the brain to the body. For an unknown reason in Multiple Sclerosis the body's immune system sees the myelin sheath as foreign and attacks it. This attack results in the breakdown of the myelin sheath, demyelination, which results in a lesion or scar on the fibre with no myelin around the nerve axon. The transfer of messages cannot occur when there is a scar on the myelin sheath and so the energy or impulse has to find another route. Eventually the number of other routes is none and the MS sufferer cannot move that part of their body. This is how the body becomes paralysed. 'Sclerosis' means scars and therefore 'Multiple Sclerosis' means many scars.

Without the insulating myelin around the nerve fibre, the nerve signals cannot pass through the cell correctly. This is supposedly where the trouble lies; if the signals cannot get through the axon then the organ receiving the signal either mixes up the message or does not receive it at all. I get a lot of pain in the left side of my arm and leg but this is just where there is a mixed message to my brain and the pain is its reaction.

Demyelination only occurs in the central nervous system with MS. The peripheral nervous system is unaffected during MS.

Who gets it?

The cause of MS is not yet known. Approximately 85,000 people living in the UK have been diagnosed with this disease. More females than males seem to come down with the illness; this is in a 3:2 ratio. The most common age to discover the illness is between the ages of 25 and 40, although I know of a case where a child was only two when they were diagnosed. MS is the most common, potentially disabling disease of the nervous system that affects young adults.

Four types of MS

There are generally four different types of MS.

1) Benign mild MS

15% of all MS sufferers have this type of MS.

There are only a few attacks.

Attacks are followed by a complete recovery.

There is no permanent disability.

This is, by far, the best case to have as the symptoms and the effects of the illness are very small.

2) Relapsing, remitting MS

70% of all MS sufferers (the majority) have this type of MS.

During the remissions there are fever/milder symptoms.

Relapses can last for an hour, a day or even a year or two.

After several attacks, the myelin damage has and will continue increasing which may allow residual damage. A sufferer will be affected more than they would have been before the attack.

I was diagnosed with this type of MS at the tender age of seventeen. Patients are often known to move onto type 4 after starting with relapsing remitting type of MS.

3) Primary progressive MS

Approximately15% or all sufferers are inflicted by this type

Sufferers start with only attacks and no remissions.

Progressive disability occurs after a relatively short period.

There are ever-worsening symptoms.

This type is potentially life threatening.

4) Secondary progressive MS

Of relapsing and remitting sufferers, 45% go into secondary progressive MS.

Begins with the relapsing, remitting MS. This will be the type of illness until remissions halt and it becomes progressive.

As MS is a disease of the central nervous system (the brain and the spinal cord) every part of the body can be affected ranging from symptoms such as eyesight issues down to pins and needles in the toes. It can affect any part of the body.

Possible symptoms of MS

MS affects each patient in a different way with no two sufferers showing exactly the same symptoms. It seems so strange that every one of the UK's 85,000 MS patients basically have their illness all to themselves!

- Vision problems
- Balance problems
- Dizziness
- Fatigue
- Bladder problems or lack of control
- Bowel problems
- Stiffness
- Spasms
- Memory problems
- Speech problems and slurring words
- Issues with swallowing
- Tremors
- Pins and needles sensation in limbs
- Pain

I personally suffer from, or have suffered from, or have experienced all of these symptoms with just the spasms and the tremors happening only after my swimming races when I need to use my wheelchair for approximately twenty minutes after each race. It is amazing that there are so many alterations of exactly the same illness! MS is pretty scary and frustrating but also pretty incredible! How can the body attack itself? Why would it go into overdrive and see itself and its own features as a bad thing? It makes me think of Stephen Spielberg's film 'AI' (Artificial Intelligence) which starred Haley Joel Osment as an android and Jude Law. In it, the android wants to be as realistic as an actual person.

I feel that if Artificial Intelligence can build computers to think for us I am certain AI can fix our body or our mind, whichever is in control of our MS. We just need to work out how!

CHAPTER 12

Life Goes On

17th June 1999
Dear Diary,
I am living a pointless life. Mum gave me a book about Multiple
Sclerosis this morning because she thinks that this is what I have. It
is awful. The book says what could or will probably happen to me
and there are awful possibilities. I am going to be useless, sitting in
a wheelchair unable to move and will lose everything I have ever
known and loved.

I don't want to be in a wheelchair. I don't want to be hand-fed or
looked after in a hospital or care home. Why has this horrid illness
attacked me? I have done everything right, why has everything gone
so very awfully wrong? At school I was the only one in my family
who didn't get sent to the headmaster or who didn't end up doing
something wrong. I did everything right, always. Why did I have to
get sick? Why is this life, my life, so wrong, so unfair?

I was getting sicker every day and the feeling of being alone was
ever-increasing. Nobody could help me now. I cried every day. Every
day and in every way. It just burst out as if I was not in any control.
I would be laughing about something and then the laughter would
turn to hot, painful tears, and then the knife in my heart would pull
me down into a sodden ball. A gut-wrenching sorrow holding me in

a knot, an enclosed and protected foetal position where I believe I could not be hurt any more.

I spent most of my spare time sitting in my room with Spring listening to sad songs because then no one could see my tears; Spring wasn't going to tell anyone. What was I supposed to do now? I had lost everything I had been so careful and so determined to work for. I had fought so hard. My life was over, or at least it might as well have been. I struggled to walk, struggled to see, struggled to move; why had it all fallen down so quickly? Everything I had taken for granted and everything anyone else would have taken for granted had given up on me and what has it left me with? Nothing. Absolutely nothing. No hope, no life. Nothing. Is there any point in me being alive anymore? Is there any point in doing all the good things that I have done all my life? If I had been a bad person maybe I wouldn't have got sick. Maybe then my life wouldn't have been forced into a wheelchair.

I suffered immense pain all down my left side with my left wrist being almost unbearable on occasions. What was I doing wrong? What was causing this pain? My ankles kept giving way by falling to the side leaving me either tripping up and desperately trying to find my balance or falling clumsily to the ground bruising every part of my body. Why had I been so good when all the bad people get away with everything? How come I don't do anything wrong and my life still goes down like a ton of bricks? Life seemed so wrong; or rather my life seemed so wrong. Why did I have to get sick? I didn't deserve it. I didn't do anything wrong. I believe in a life for a life, or at least, if you do something wrong you should get punishment for it! Again, I don't deserve this. I didn't do anything wrong.

CHAPTER 13

Disability Appeal

Stephanie Millward
Box,
Corsham
Wilts

10th October 2000

Dear Disability Living Allowance People,

I was very pleased when I received your letter of 26th September that stated I wasn't entitled to a Disability Living Allowance.

Does this mean that I am not disabled?

Does this mean that I can once again start my career as an Olympic Swimming hopeful?

Does this mean that my memory has once again come back and I can re-sit my A-levels and this time pass?

Does this mean that I can go to university or perhaps get a good job?

Does this mean that I can once again go shopping for more than a few brief minutes?

Does this mean that I can walk more than 100 metres?

Does this mean that I won't keep falling down?
Does this mean that I have a real life?

It would be GREAT but I suspect that the above isn't true and that I am, as it is so quaintly called, disabled.

It means that I can't swim and get out of a swimming pool without someone watching my progress up the steps then helping me to totter across the floor.

It means that my habit of writing lists helps compensate for my lack of memory. Now, if I could just remember where I put those lists.

It means that I'll never go to university, even though I did fail maths, biology and economics, and as for a job, well, there's about as much success there as I have had from the Disability Living Allowance People.

It means that I don't go shopping unless it's really vital and my mum is free to come with me – thank goodness for mail order.

It means that I still can't walk more than 100 metres without having to sit (or fall) down.

It means that I can still expect other mishaps to go with the two falls on my face this month.

It means a life with Multiple Sclerosis.

Please explain why I did not qualify; I do not understand.
What does it mean to be disabled?
Why am I not classified as disabled?

I want to appeal.

Yours sincerely,
Stephanie

CHAPTER 14

Giving Up, 18th June 1999

I told my mum that I needed a wheelchair today because I'd had enough of struggling to walk, looking for something to hold all the time. The shocked look on her face sent the inside of my heart hurriedly doing somersaults. She didn't want me to have one and obviously I really didn't want one but on this occasion I would have to let the MS win. I have had enough of getting into Bath and being unable to go anywhere.

I remember one time while I was in Bath on my own I was stood leaning against a fence hoping that someone would come and offer me their arm to lean on or perhaps get me a seat for a minute. I was standing in the car park with my car sat approximately ten metres away from me but my legs just stopped working and there was no hand rail between this fence and my car, just open ground. I saw people looking at me wondering why someone so young was struggling but obviously they couldn't help me, they were too busy. They had a life to lead, I was too sick for anyone to care about. They didn't need to help me. I'll stand here leaning against the wall feeling sorry for myself and hoping again that 'God' would send someone to help. He didn't.

After waiting for a while leaning against the fence I started moving slowly. Right foot first, inch it forward. I felt as though I was walking on a trapeze trying to get my balance. Inch by inch I moved towards my car, the goal post and my safety net. Stop for a break, deep breath, another step. Inside the car I have no limitations. Nobody can see my pain and they definitely can't see how far I can walk. They would never know that I am sick. Inside the car I can be whoever I want to be. As long as there is petrol in the car I can go wherever I want to go. I can be free. Outside of the car I have to control these legs that obviously don't want to work for me. Outside is a whirlpool where anything could happen. Everything I used to take for granted is punching me in the face now, paying me back for not appreciating it before. Maybe this is what I did wrong? Maybe I didn't say thank you for every wonderful thing I had been given at birth?

Thankfully, now that I have been awarded a disabled badge (after my letter was received) I can to park closer to the shops which means a shorter distance to walk. Come on, Stephanie. Inch by inch, you can do it!

I eventually reached my gold mine and sat in my car taking deep breaths of relief. I had worked so hard to get here today I was exhausted. The little blue Metro was my true companion. Reliably sitting there waiting for me, it never disobeyed my orders, it never complained, it never let me down. I wish my legs were as dependable.

I was advised to go see a physio who I saw a few times. She gave me a walking stick to help with my balance. A large brown walking stick that elderly people used; I can't use one of those. The stick looked awful when it was anywhere near me and I hated it. I can't walk around with this ugly monster no way. I don't need a stick; I am still a child, or a young adult anyway! Even my granny doesn't need a stick. Maybe I could chop it in half and throw it for a dog? Maybe I could set it on fire? I can walk by the walls and the wall can be my stick. I don't need a stick.

I often had this inability to walk and it annoyed me that nobody ever tried to help. I suppose nobody knew how much I was hurting or how much I had lost. This was my fight and my war and I would have to learn to fight it on my own.

No cause, no cure. Absolutely, completely and utterly no hope.

CHAPTER 15

Fatigue

The disability appeal letter worked and a doctor was sent to my house to watch me manoeuvre up the hill. After asking if I could stop for a break after only about six metres I was allowed to go home and put my feet up. The doctor didn't even need to test my legs or make me walk further; he saw the distress and pain in my eyes. He knew I was living a lie and fighting it with every step. The doctor must have known that I could not take too much more and thankfully for me I was given the label 'disabled'. I hated being seen as disabled and hated the word with all my might but I knew that my perfect life was in the past now and that I had to come to terms with this new title - Stephanie Millward, the girl with MS who receives benefits because she is disabled. Ouch! This may take some time to come to terms with. I was the perfect girl living the perfect life. For sixteen years I had perfection and I will always be thankful of that. The other however many number of years I will be paying the price for something I am not even certain I did wrong. At least I had sixteen wonderful years!

I later swapped my trusty blue Metro for a Renault Clio on the Motability scheme. I was thrilled with the new car and impressed with the Motability deal that was awarded to me for being disabled! You can swap your Disability Living Allowance payments for a car. The insurance for two people is paid by the allowance and the car tax is also free as it is part of the deal! What a wonderful help - all this made my life a little bit easier!

I also had a new feeling which was a symptom, an excuse and a nightmare all at the same time - fatigue. Fatigue is not the same as tiredness, it is a form of or an inability to do something or anything; I could not move because my legs felt laden down with coal and bricks. Nothing wanted to move. People keep saying they are tired. Wow, they really have no idea what real tiredness feels like. Able-bodied swimmers with nothing wrong complain they are tired. If only they could feel a tiny bit of what I am feeling, just a tiny bit would shock them for a life time and they would never say, 'I am so tired', again. The inability to move your arms or legs just because of pure fatigue and the dead weight of muscles that just don't want to move - how can anyone compare? If only they knew! Ignorance is bliss but I suppose you can only comment on what you know or something you have experienced. I have now experienced both forms of tiredness: the normal person's tired and the MS person's tired. 100% different. With the normal person's tired you can still move. With the MS person's tired (fatigue) you might as well be strapped to the ground by lead ropes; you need to fight through this burden just to be able to move a millimetre.

From the moment you get up in the morning to the last thing at night all you have is the constant feeling of exhaustion, having to stop for breaks to ensure you don't over tire yourself. It was almost like a game of cat and mouse - trying to push myself as much as I could but not letting the MS catch up.

Muscle strength is also affected as a side effect to fatigue. This is also known as 'MS Lassitude' (that's what my doctor said!). Fatigue can cause inactivity and muscle weakness (like I said, being strapped to the floor with little or no relief). Muscle atrophy can also be caused by a lack of movement due to balance or gait issues as well as dizziness (vertigo); all of which are symptoms of MS and all a bit of a nuisance from my point of view.

Another problem I struggled with was that the inflammation on my brain severely affected my short-term memory and every name or even the things on my 'to do list' were forgotten as soon as I had thought them up. It was very frustrating and I ended up writing Post-it notes to remind me to do everything. My A-levels, unfortunately, were never going to be easy with the lack of memory and the eyesight issues stopped everything but, still believing I could do anything, I kept going to school and kept trying to relearn the information. If I could move everything into my long-term memory maybe I could remember it. Unfortunately, my long-term memory was affected too with the stress of getting the MS, and my exams were another very disappointing affair.

Looking back at this, wondering if I could have done anything differently, I feel that now I would try to use my long-term memory more and spend longer on each subject to make sure that I remembered it. I think that my A-level exams were just something for me that came perhaps at the wrong time when I was still trying to find my place in the world and with the new addition of a disease nobody knew anything about!

Getting the diagnosis for MS was a relief as it was a name for the symptoms I was experiencing and it was something to blame. I believe that everything happens for a reason and I kept looking at everything I had done in my life; I wondered why I had been selected the illness when in my eyes I had done nothing to deserve it. I had always been hard-working and determined and never bad. I didn't think therefore that this was a reaction from something I had done. Maybe God had given me MS to give other people strength. Maybe if I can be someone that people look up to and find inspiring it would make the MS that much easier?

Maybe I got MS so that I can give people hope? Yeah, maybe, as this is a very worthwhile reason! I have to experience all the MS symptoms so I know what other people are feeling.

OK, MS. Hit me with anything! I am ready! I am doing it for the MS population!

CHAPTER 16

Blind

I was standing in the kitchen with Spring in my arms when I first went blind, aged just seventeen. My eyesight just went, all of it. The colours, the sun, the light, everything just disappeared and it was instead replaced by a black hole. I could see nothing out of either eye and the fear that rose inside me was immense. I started crying. What is happening to me? Am I going to be able to see again? Am I going to be blind forever? Have I caused this? Why have I gone blind? Again, what did I do wrong?

I sat down because at least the floor would not move and I felt quite safe there. Spring licked my hand.

'Mum? Mum, I can't see!' The tears were coming out hard and fast as if trying to use water power to push the black blanket away.

'Mum...'

'Don't worry, it will all be fine.' I could feel her strength beside me. 'It will come back, you will be OK.'

I felt very lonely in this black little world of mine and wondered how people survived being blind. I felt sorry for everyone who was unfortunate enough to have lost their eyesight and I felt sorry for myself now. Is it all going to come back or have I lost it forever? Am I ever going to be able to see again? Spring, my constant companion, licked my hand again making me smile. The tears stopped flowing and I tried to relax and get some control back on my life. Putting Spring on the ground I got up.

'Can you see yet?' asked my mum.

Shaking my head I put my hand out to try to find out where I was. I had a mental picture of the kitchen in my mind and I tried to feel my way to the counter where the kettle sat. Picking the kettle up to see if there is any water in it I felt the weight signifying that there was no water inside. I was looking for some comfort which I would find in the cup of tea! I sighed and started thinking about being like this forever.

'I will fill it up.' My mum took the kettle out of my hands and moved to the sink. If I am going to be like this forever my mum will have to take that role of looking after me. She will be my carer as well as my mother. I can't ruin her life like that.

Thankfully, my eyesight came back a little bit later and the feeling of relief was extreme. I was very thankful that I was back to normal and that I didn't have to remain blind forever. Will I go blind again or is that it? Is MS going to steal my eyesight for good eventually? About a week later I lost my eyesight again. This time I felt more confident as I knew my eyesight was going to come back eventually. I mean, it did last time so it should do this time. The period of time it took seemed like forever and I could almost hear the clock ticking the seconds away. Finally, after the ten or fifteen minutes were up the alarm sounded silently and the colours were back. I appreciate colours, pictures and photos far more now than ever before and the sun always deserves a smile when it is showing us its beautiful face!

In total I lost my eyesight three times with the length of time being blind increasing on each occasion. Every time my mum was strong for me and every time Spring was there beside me like a cuddly toy comforting me and helping to keep me going. I have a silent appreciation for my eyesight and whenever my sight trembles I worry that this may be the time when I will lose it forever. Who knows when or if I will go blind forever? My MS makes this possibility more likely. Does anyone else go blind at seventeen? I am sure they do but what an awful possibility. Colours bring with them a silent warmth and a comfort that I suppose you only appreciate after a long, dark winter. Even so, the sun is always exciting, signalling the start of spring or summer and the indication of summer holidays and the excitement they bring.

Going blind has taught me a number of lessons about appreciation and desire. I am always happy when the wonderful sun is shining and I thank God for the ability to see the colours. Colourful paintings have taken on a new desire in my life and I find artists and their paintings very important. Maybe my eyesight went so that I could learn to appreciate all the things that the blindness took away. I know my eyesight may go again, maybe for longer or even forever, so I have come to terms with the fact that one day I may need to get a guide dog to show me where to go. This is a lovely thought even with the obvious ramifications. I met a lovely couple who train guide dogs as puppies and they told me all about the amazing things guide dogs can help their owner with. This knowledge has left me feeling more confident with the thought that going blind is not the end of the earth, just the start of a new way of life. Even though being blind is a scary thought I know I am now strong enough to keep going through anything with or without my eyesight!

CHAPTER 17

Nicholas, aka Mister

I don't really know why I call him Mister but I do remember that it has something to do with a certain 'Mister Nu' while a youngster! Mister has stuck with him and in exchange he calls me Step.

With Paul as an unbeatable monster truck, me as a winning Ferrari and Kristy as a fashionable Beetle Convertible, Nicholas had to follow a good lead and in some ways I feel sorry for him. I would still put him as a stretch limo where he would have a chauffeur driving him around while he would lounge around and spend all his time chatting to his friends! Mister was still very young when we left Saudi Arabia and moved to England which I feel is a shame as I cherish my memories of Saudi Arabia. Maybe one day we can all return to Jeddah safely and welcome the sights and sounds from our childhoods. When we were young, Mister was my best friend, my companion, always by my side. We did everything together and we really enjoyed each other's company.

Mister read many books learning in his own way about history, about life, about make believe. Every time I looked over at him he was finishing yet another different book! Academically Nicholas was probably the cleverest of the four of us but possibly before he had the chance to home in on something he would do for the rest of his life, the focus turned to me because I was sick. For Nicholas it must have been a huge shock. This seemed to change his perspective on life and he wanted, or possibly needed, to try anything and everything to see what he wanted to do in life. I had always been a great source of knowledge, determination, strength and hope so when I got sick it affected Mister the most. The strength he used to find in me started wilting and eventually it ebbed away.

Nicholas is gradually coming to terms with my MS and is learning to deal with it in his own way. Mister is very gifted with his words and I believe he will one day be a wonderful author, philosophising about life through his beautiful thoughts and stunning words. Mister can communicate to anyone and this ability will be fantastic for him. He is also incredibly caring and even when I saw the pain through his eyes I knew that once the onset of my illness had settled down in our minds, he would be a good friend again. He just needed to come to terms with the unfairness part of life, the why-did-Stephanie-have-to-get-sick part, the will-it-happen-to-me bit of this equation. Nicholas is lovely and caring and always looks to make someone smile. When completely broke he will spend his last few pennies buying his friends drinks!

I hope Nicholas will be around me forever so that we can regain that pure trust and love and we can be friends and play again as we did while we were young. He was and still is the cute baby brother that we don't ever want to grow up! We will cherish our friendship forever.

CHAPTER 18
Paralysed

'Help! Help! Help! Help me, please. Help... me... please!' I was screaming and tears were falling down my face.

'Please!' I tried to move anything but I couldn't. My body lay still, ignoring my every request. Legs? No. Arms? Face? What?

'Please, please, please. Pretty please!' I don't even know who I was crying to or what I was screaming for. I knew the house was empty.

'Please!' Maybe God could come down to save me. I was desperate for the toilet but was stuck lying on my back in bed. I had woken in a state of paralysis and there was no way I could get to the bathroom.

'Help!' I screamed again almost realising I may have to go here in my bed. I thought I had been in charge of the MS as it had been good for a few days. I had even walked to work! Why has it all changed now? I haven't done anything wrong. The big question again, 'Why me?' I could hear Spring's cries and scratching on the back of the door. She was trying to help me but obviously her thirty-centimetre size limited the ways she could help. I wanted her next to me for comfort but there was no way of letting her in. I took a deep breath, trying to get more strength.

Move the feet, right foot first. This is the stronger one.

'Move!' I yelled the familiar word viciously as though the voice would cause vibrations to move the foot.

'Move, flaming move!' I was desperately searching for anything that could help me.

'WWRRRRAAAAAAHHH!' The anger and frustration came out loud and strong and I felt the heart broken sobs where my whole body motionless was screaming with pain.

'Mum, Dad, Paul, Kristy, MISTER? Help me, please. Someone, anyone please help!' I screamed one last time before realising my precious time was just about up.

'Oh...' I sighed realising that this illness was far more unexpected and cruel than I had first imagined. I had read the book my mum gave me from front to back and had realised that there are many horrible symptoms of MS and that wetting the bed was just one of the minor ones. However minor, I didn't want this to be my first time.

'Help?' I try again hoping someone had magically entered the house without making any noise. 'HELP! Please, please, please help me. Please.' I don't want to lose. Not now, not ever. 'Please help me.'

Trying to move seemed almost unreal. I have been moving freely for seventeen years; why has it all stopped now? I had never done anything wrong, I don't deserve this.

'Help?' Do I just go to the toilet here? Is anyone going to help me? Sighing again I shut my eyes and a tear fell to my cheek. Don't start crying now, Stephanie, I told myself. Stay in control, stay strong. 'Mum? Kristy? Anyone?' I was losing hope and time was running out. 'Please?'

Then, as if a dream had been answered, I heard a key turn in the front door. Yes yes yes! There was light at the end of the tunnel!

'Help! Help! Help! Help! Help!' I started the familiar yell, feeling that there may be someone to save me. It seemed a very long time before I heard the handle being pulled down.

'Please!' A wail that held every emotion possible. 'Please help!'

Nicholas came into the room closely followed by Spring.

'What's wrong?' he asked with concern all over his face. Spring jumped on the bed and started kissing me to dry the tears.

'I can't move and I need to go to the toilet,' I said and the relieved tears came flooding down my face.

In a commanding tone Nicholas said, 'Don't worry, I will help.'

He grabbed my legs and pulled them to the side of the bed. Then, grasping both of my hands in one of his hands, he put an arm under my neck to keep it stable. He then pulled my arms over his neck. Bending his knees he pulled me up off the bed.

'Hold on', he said and I tried with all my might.

Nicholas all but dragged me to the toilet where I sat exhausted but thankful.

Nicholas was my saviour. He had saved me from a certain disaster. I love my brother, he is unbeatable and I will remember that moment for the rest of my life!

Sometimes I feel that God is testing us to the limit to see how much we can take. I had kept strong in the belief that God would get someone to come into the house to help me even though it had seemed like a hopeless dream. But before I had given up he did answer my prayer. If I had given up straight away it would have had awful consequences but the trust in God and in life's coincidences had meant that I could keep the belief going and then the magic happened with my brother coming home at just the right moment. Truly incredible!

Coincidences, I believe, happen for a reason as though our life story has already been mapped out for us and the coincidences happen sometimes just to get us back on track! Life is still such an amazing creation and we are so lucky!

CHAPTER 19

Steroids, 12th June 2000

Dear Diary,

My life has changed completely and not for the better. I am sitting AS-level exams while on steroids. How am I meant to do well in my exams when I am constantly thinking about my probable illness and about the steroids which are being put into my body intravenously every day? How am I meant to do well when the things I have taken for granted, such as my eyes, are not doing their jobs correctly and I am left with somebody reading me the questions? Am I supposed to do as well as everyone else even though my body is giving up and I am dripping with my own tears and every part of my body is crying out in pain?

Why am I sick now? It could have waited until after my exams and after the Olympics. I could have got sick when I was a proper age, not seventeen and still a child. What did I do so wrong? I had such a perfect life. Maybe I am now living someone else's life? This can't be happening to me.

I am going to school to take my exams but somewhere inside me I know I will fail them all. I feel that my whole body is testing me to the ultimate level and all I want to do is bury my head somewhere, let everyone forget I was ever alive, and then one day I could just swim out to sea and die.

I have tried to cut myself again today with the scissors. I feel almost proud when I cause myself this pain, like I have achieved something at last! I could take too many tablets but then if someone saw me I would be rushed to hospital where I would have to throw up. I hate throwing up. I feel that the pain of the scissors digging into me is much better than throwing up. The blood caused by the scissors is almost a reward for the work I had been doing and the picture produced on my stomach proof that I can still do something. The pain of the scissors makes me feel stronger and more alive. The ache caused by MS is a different pain than the scissors so therefore I can forget all about that for a while. I can still be in control, I can cause the pain and therefore it is there for a reason, I can be in charge!

Why did I have to get sick at seventeen? I feel like I am still a baby. Why couldn't I have been like everyone else and passed their exams and then gone on to university where I would meet a partner, get married and have a baby? The normal life story. Why am I so different? Why did my life have to get hit with an illness? Why did I have to lose all my dreams and why is the Olympic dream over before it even began? Why am I left here, a discarded lump of fat with no useful life left to live? None of the days I am living are worth the hours the clock is ticking. I just don't understand why am I sick now? Why couldn't it have waited? Why am I living a dead-end life? There is no need for me now. I am sick. I deserve to die.

During my AS-level exams I was sent to the hospital to be connected to a drip for a number of hours every day. The steroids made me feel very sick and very ill and my weight piled on. I was getting more and more depressed as the drugs made me feel so sick and I didn't manage to remember any of the things I had revised for in the exams anyway. My memory was giving up on me and I felt that I had nothing left. Was all this really worth it?

I returned to the doctors after my bout of steroids only to be told that the steroids hadn't worked. I had put on weight for no reason. I felt that I had let everyone down and had an illness I would have to cope with for the rest of my life. What an exciting prospect. My mum had given me that book about MS and it said the only safe stabiliser when the sufferer was sick with MS was a bout of steroids. If they didn't work for me that meant that there is no safety net for me. Nothing to help at all. If I get sick with MS there will be nothing left to help me. Nothing at all can help me now. Me against the MS. What do I get to make this a fair fight? Nobody knows anything about MS except that steroids help most people. Why on earth am I not one of those lucky ones? Don't I have any safety nets? Me against the MS. Again, I felt very lonely, like I was in it on my own forever. No one will feel my pain. I might as well give up now. I will end up in a wheelchair being fed by my mum anyway which I suppose is where I started when I was a baby. It might as well end there too. What a nightmare and what a miserable end to all my wonderful dreams. Where did I go so wrong?

The MS against me (all on my own). One nil to the MS.
 I need to make this fair or just give up on my fight.
What can give me powers?

MS Multiple Sclerosis
SM Stephanie Millward
MS SM
What a cruel joke.

CHAPTER 20

Absolutely No Control, 10th October 2000

Dear Diary

I have always taken everything for granted. Never once did I realise how special my eyesight or my ability to talk or walk was. I didn't think once how important each of these abilities was until they were no longer there, until they no longer performed in the way that they always had done for the past seventeen years. Just imagine having everything but not knowing how wonderful it all was until it was gone.

I do regret now not realising how fantastic my life was and how amazing our bodies are. I do also regret not knowing or believing that I could have anything I wanted. Now it may be a little limited but only moderately. I can do anything if I try hard enough. I am sure I can.

The MS started with my eyesight - 'optic neuritis', whatever that is - and balance problems. These symptoms reminded me of being very drunk and having no control on your arms, legs or balance. The symptoms stayed but then I went completely black-blind for short periods of time. The MS seemed to be totally in charge of what I was doing. If 'it' was having a bad day then I was having a bad day. The eyesight moved on to complete paralysis where my whole body ignored every request I made of it. I was obviously getting worried. What is going to happen to me? Will I be going in and out of these MS attacks for the rest of my life?

My bladder was the next thing to ignore my requests; I wet myself on a number of occasions. It is incredibly embarrassing when you don't even know you are going to the toilet and end up with the liquid running down your leg. Imagine being in a crowd of friends and realising that you have wet yourself. There was no control at all and I didn't even know I needed to go to the toilet. This symptom took away all my self-confidence. Imagine having absolutely no control of your everyday jobs like going to the toilet. I felt awful. My life was a complete mess.

The next embarrassing moment was the complete opposite when I felt that I was desperate for the toilet. I was rushing to find the nearest toilet, pushing in the queue because I was so desperate but then not being able to go. What a strange moment. I walked out into the large queue and I had to apologise profusely because I had been so eccentric and didn't even need the toilet in the end. I have never blushed so much in my life. My five foot seven frame shrank to mere centimetres.

MS annoyed me because I didn't have any idea what was going to happen next. I had similar problems with my bowel as I had with my bladder, each as catastrophic as the last. I ended up wanting to either stay in my room all day just in case my body ignored my requests or to kill myself, ending these uncertain fears. In my mind it would have been better to have been dead and not have to put up with these embarrassing situations then to have to worry about possible consequences every minute of my life. My mum was always very strong for me and she often helped me clear up the mess and wipe away my tears. When everything you have always taken for granted disappears you are left with nothing and the dark empty feeling is the loneliest possible moment you could ever imagine. The fact that things you have known since you were a baby go against all of your beliefs and all of your dreams. The dark tunnel opens and you are pushed inside. There is no visible way out and the ground starts sloping downwards.

I was very depressed and when my mum offered me a meeting with a psychiatrist I grasped it with open arms. Somebody, anybody please help me. Get me out of this black hole.

I went to see the psychiatrist and she listened to my every word. I finished a non-stop forty minutes of tears and forcing my words out before she said, 'You have had a hard time. Imagine you have died and are in the grieving process but will soon be over this and then you can get on with your new life.'

A new life? I thought, I don't want a new life. I want my old life, the one I was leading before because that had been wonderful. I don't want to die and then have to invent a new person. I liked me. I liked being in charge of my life and I liked knowing what my body was going to do. I didn't want a new life.

After many trips to see the psychiatrist I started understanding why I had to die in order for me to get better. I had MS for the rest of my life and so all I had to do was to try to come to terms with this and then start rebuilding my life, to pick up all my shattered pieces. I grew strong in this period of time and I realised that if I keep the pain inside nobody else gets hurt. I also got used to the pain in my left hand and arm and I started trying to use my hand more even through the pain. This meant that I could hide it without anyone else having to know I was hurting.

My eyesight caused a little more trouble with the continuous jumping and blurry double vision. I often watched TV with my family but on many occasions I couldn't make out what was happening on the screen. I pretended that I was enjoying the show but really I couldn't see anything and I was only enjoying the company of my family. At least twice a day I walked into a door or the wall; I would misjudge where I was and my eyesight just didn't work well enough to see where I was going. This still happens now and I walk into the edge of a wall or door where I have not seen the distance quite well enough. Going down stairs I can't see that the second step is lower than the first. This is quite a dangerous problem but I have got used to watching what the person in front of me does and I therefore know if there is a step coming up. Looking through the negative parts of my illness I see now how I can be called disabled even though I look exactly the same as I did when I was considered to be able.

I think 'disability' is described by having 'absolutely no control' on some or all parts of your body. I now consider myself to be a little bit disabled but hopefully this disability won't get any worse and that I will remain mildly disabled for the rest of my life.

I used to get stupidly drunk so that I could forget all my problems. Maybe one day after getting very drunk I will be reborn without the MS, without the sore arm, without the bladder issues. Maybe this alcohol will have a chemical reaction with my MS and make me all better again. Maybe I will just wake up and realise that this part of my life was just a bad dream. Getting so drunk whenever I went out, I think, was a reaction to my depression. I needed to be worried about something else for a change; my illness was no longer the main thing on my mind as the drink took over and I didn't care about what would happen. I didn't mind if I fell over when I was drunk as this is what you are meant to do; the drink makes you fall and, happily, you get back up again. With the MS it drags you down and you have to fight with yourself to even think about getting back up. The tension in your face is not a smile and laughter but instead is a grimace of disgust and you have lost again. The MS is in charge; you are down and have absolutely no control. The illness is in control. The MS, on this occasion, has won.

CHAPTER 21

The Failings

Well, where do I start? I have failed at everything in life and I am left with absolutely nothing. The Olympic Games in Sydney this year (2000) was supposed to be my year, my Games. I was meant to win the races and come out on top as the golden girl shining in every light on every stage and loving the whole atmosphere; this was my life story. The media were making a big thing of the Games by supporting everything about it and the team. The best Games ever, apparently! The whole country was excited about this competition but in my house nobody paid it any attention and nobody spoke about it. A broken dream for me that my family tried to protect.

I knew when the team were flying to Sydney, I knew where the holding camp was and I knew everything about the Olympic site. I was meant to be on that team. I was supposed to fly out there with them to compete. It was my dream too. Instead, I sat in my room with Spring unable to even switch on the TV to support the team. The thought of the Games and my seat on that plane made me cry and cry again and again. That was my Olympic Games.

I failed all of my AS-level exams in the year 2000, the year I was meant to shine. There was no point doing these exams as I got nothing from going through the stress and anxiety caused by them. The exam papers were read to me by a school helper and I was given an extra fifteen minutes in case I needed more time. These little things seemed incredibly futile and the teachers may as well have said to me: You are going to fail anyway so we will isolate you from the rest of the school and then read the questions to you. They were just trying to be helpful, but I felt very stupid. I felt humiliated and made to feel like a baby. I am eighteen years old, I am neither stupid nor a baby. They might as well have shot me down. I used to be so clever but now am left with this? Horrendous.

All the pupils went back to Corsham School one morning to collect their exam results for our AS-level exams. I didn't know what to expect. Opening the letter labelled 'Stephanie Millward Exam Results' had felt like listening to a judge telling me whether I was going to be given a life in prison or was going to be given another chance. The results were obviously the former option and it just made me cry again. My sister Kristy had also received her letter which had awarded her a very successful set of GCSE results. I had turned my back on everyone and was walking away from all the excited students who were laughing and giggling. I just wanted to die. I had done all the revision so I knew all the work; how did I get nothing except a big fat fail? Maybe if I walked onto the road someone would run me over. Maybe I would just die and then no one will have to find out my marks. No one would have to listen to me speak or have to pick me up if I fall again. They will all be better off without me. I have to get away. I have to go. No one can help me. I am useless. Rubbish.

'Stephanie, we are going to the pub for a drink. Would you like to come?' my mum asked.

Does it look like I want to go to the pub? I had been awarded all fails, what would I want to celebrate about that? I have failed I am useless. Actually, maybe I can drink too much alcohol which will kill me. I must have make-up all down my face from my tears.

'Stephanie?' My mum was right beside me and had put an arm around my shoulder in her caressing way. 'I can take you home if you wish but you might feel better if you have a quick drink.'

This was the start of my covering-ups. I told everyone I hadn't done quite as well as expected and needed to work harder to get the A-level exam results that I wanted.

On one occasion, soon after the exam results, I had gone to the doctors where I asked for an urgent appointment. I was given a session and while I was sat in the waiting room I felt like a convict. Everyone kept looking at me as though I had done something wrong. When I walked into the doctor's room I sat down and cried. The pain throughout my body was extreme and everything hurt. It took me, what felt like, about an hour to stop crying and then the doctor asked if I was OK. Stupid question really. She started me on antidepressants; two a day for the first week and then I was to return for another appointment. I went home and took five tablets. Maybe these could help me? Maybe they could kill me? I read the little leaflet that came with the tablets: 'Do not exceed the stated dose'. Yep, it could kill me. The tablets helped me to sleep and this was a benefit as at last I stopped crying. I slept for the whole night and woke the next day with almost a smile on my face.

I took Spring for a walk just up the road. I was enjoying the sun which shone wonderfully in the sky and I was thinking about going up to the shop and buying an ice cream. Yes, what a good idea. I told Spring what I was going to do and I think she agreed that it was a brilliant idea. We started our walk but, like a lightning bolt from the sky, I could feel the pain all down my leg just before it fell sideways, bringing me down with it. What? I had such nice feelings and expectations for this walk why has it hit me again? I steadied myself to try to get up and with a huge push from my arms I managed to stand. What do I do now? I phoned my mum and asked her to come and get me which she did. My mum was used to coming to save the day for me and never once did I think about her. It was a day a few days later when I was sat eating my dinner when my mum asked 'How are you getting on with the antidepressants?'

How does she know I am on antidepressants? 'Huh?' was my remark.

'I went to the doctor and got antidepressants for myself and the doctor mentioned it.'

'Oh.' She's on antidepressants because of me. I have made somebody so upset that they have to get medication.

'Sorry,' I said.

'It's not your fault', she said.

But it was.

I continued on the tablets as they were supposed to make me feel happier. They didn't really so when I visited the doctor a week later I asked her why and she replied that they need longer to work. I decided to have one large amount of the antidepressants to see if they made me feel better so I took ten before I fell asleep. The next day I woke up later than normal and I was in a bad mood. I started moaning about everything and cried on a number of occasions. The overdose didn't help at all. I went back to the normal two-tablets-a-day dose and decided that I needed a job to try to do something in this life of mine. I went to the Co-operative shop up the road and they accepted my CV. They invited me for an interview which I went to with a smile on my face. I might be better than useless if I can start earning some money. I was given a job which I loved doing. All I had to do was fill the shelves, tidy the shop and serve the customers. This job gave me a wonderful sense of achievement and I always felt excited about the next day at work. It is a shame that this relatively easy life didn't stay so simple.

A whole year later Kristy and I went to Tenerife with some of Kristy's friends. I hoped I would be well on this trip but instead I forgot some of my injections, had my purse and all my money stolen, struggled with the MS and Kristy and I just fought the whole time - she had obviously given up being nice about my mood swings and my bad temperedness. It's fair enough really, looking back at it. While we were away Kristy was meant to receive her AS-level results and I was meant to receive my A-level results. I was worried sick. I had failed all my AS-level exams so I was worried that I would have the same results this time. My mum had to go and collect the results and she read them to us over the phone. Stephanie, you have done quite well: an E for biology and two Ns (nearly) for economics and maths. What? Fail, fail and an even bigger, fatter fail. I felt so sick. This wasn't meant to happen.

Kristy spoke to mum after me. Kristy had received a B grade for the AS-level exam she had done in biology. It felt as though she had sprinkled salt in to my cuts to make them hurt more. Why did I have to get sick? I was the clever one in the family. Kristy was the fashion person. I was the brains. Why did she have to get the grade that I should have got? I got nothing. I obviously wasn't going to go to university this year because I wasn't good enough. Other people were going to have a year out too so it seemed a viable excuse but I wasn't EVER going to go to University. I failed.I had also failed at swimming and so had to hear the adverts on the TV telling of the amazing Sydney 2000 Olympic Games. Apparently the firework displays had been wonderful and all the athletes had competed well. I should have been there. I should have gone to Australia with the team. I was good enough; I should have gone. Instead I had sat in my room with my little dog crying. I hadn't watched the Olympics as it had felt too painful and it had stirred too many sorrowful images in my mind. Their joy should have been my joy. I should have swum well in my first Olympics. I should have celebrated afterwards. I should have gone to the first Olympics of the new century.

Why was it all so rudely ripped away from me? Why had my life been left in such a shattered mess? I asked these two questions many times wondering the huge question, 'Why me?' If I had believed in God a little more would I have got MS? Maybe it was my fault, then, as I never go to church. This must be the reason. Or maybe the devil is playing a nasty trick on me to see if I do believe in God or maybe he or it just wants me to go to hell to live in misery with him. Maybe in a former life I killed somebody and am therefore going to pay for it in this lifetime. Maybe I deserve it.

These thoughts ran through my mind many times during a day and I started believing that I deserved it and that I therefore had to put up with all the nasty things because I had been so awful in another life. It was my fault and I must therefore pay for it. Spring stayed beside me all the time and as a companion I couldn't have asked for a better source of comfort. She was loving all day and all night. She was my angel who was probably sent from God to go through this awful time with me. I wrote a large number of poems, many of which

CHAPTER 22

Judy!

'Hi!' Judy said walking into the Co-op and seeing me serving behind the till.

'Hi ya! How are you?'

'Yeah, I'm good! I ride horses once a week in Bradford on Avon in a disabled group. Would you like to come with me?' Judy asked.

Wow! I haven't been on a horse for years but I have always loved them; I wonder how good I will be now with the MS.

I wasn't good, and again the MS was completely in charge of all of my limbs and my balance. I needed help to get on the horse in the first place and Thistle the grey horse I was riding looked at me as though I was stupid. I had ridden Thistle many times when I was younger but it all seemed so much harder now. We walked round the ménage first and my confidence increased a little but when the instructor asked for a trot I had a sharp reminder that I was no longer 'able'. Thistle had quite a bouncy trot and as she began to move faster I was hoisted sideways and sat strangely on the saddle. Thistle started moving away from the side of the riding school and slowed down to a walk. She was completely in control and I was just a useless lump sat on a bored horse in the middle of the ring.

The instructor asked one of her helpers to lead Thistle round so that I could concentrate on my balance without having to think about where Thistle was going. This helped a lot and riding became easier. I was eventually allowed to control the horse on my own again and we started concentrating on basic dressage skills. Judy was very good at riding even though she had to have to have one of her legs amputated because of cancer, but she had no issues with balance! Judy was a great inspiration to me.

Judy came to my house every Monday to pick me up for riding. We chatted happily on the drive there and then were even more excited after the ride. Judy told me all about her wonderful family with her four children and I told her about my life as a swimmer and then getting sick. Judy explained that she had to have her leg amputated when she got cancer in it. This was a shock as I didn't think anyone else got sick, just me. This was a reminder that I was just a pawn in the game of life and I started thinking more about other people and what they were doing in their lives and how they were feeling. Judy taught me a lot about attitudes to disabled people and about life as a disabled person. She was very strong.

There was a guy who rode with us and he always grinned at us when we went horse riding but he was very disabled and needed help with every part of riding. I decided to find out what was wrong with him. Judy smiled nicely at me before saying, 'Stephanie, he has progressive MS.' It felt as though someone had kicked me in the stomach. Am I going to be like that when I am older? The doctors had always said that I got MS very young and that I will be in a wheelchair by my fifth year of having MS. Will I have progressive MS before I am twenty? This is not fair.

The friendship between Judy and I increased and I depended on her strength every time I saw her. I was so proud to know her. On the drive to riding one day we were talking and Judy said that if she got cancer again she would die. Of course I jumped in and said, 'No way. You are well now. You are not going to get cancer again'.

But the doubt was there. I should have known when she had even mentioned it that something was wrong. Judy called me up a few weeks later and said that she couldn't ride that week because she didn't feel very well. The week after she said that she was very sorry but she wouldn't be able to ride again ever. She had got cancer again.

Why did she have to get sick? She was such a nice person and so young. I visited Judy at her house every day and I saw her deteriorate rapidly. After seeing her I would go home and cry. Life is so cruel. Judy died of cancer as she had foreseen and the loss in my heart was extreme. I prayed to God and asked all the questions. Why do people die? Why did she die so young? She had cancer once before, surely you could have given it to someone else?

Judy's funeral was jam-packed with her friends. I cried loudly the whole way through it. I was distraught and didn't know how to control the tears. This was the first time I had lost a friend through death. What a pain-filled experience.

I appreciate all the wonderful things Judy did for me. She offered me hope which I grasped with both hands. In her own way she was a guardian angel and I will remember her fondly forever.

Thank you, Judy, for everything!

CHAPTER 23

The Drug – Beta Interferon B

There is one drug, the one chance left for me. This is the drug Beta Interferon type B. Beta Interferon is an interferon drug that gets inserted into the body's immune system using an injection. I have always had a fear of needles and the only drug available to me was an injection! Why is life so mean? I have always felt very sorry for any sufferers of diabetes who have to inject insulin into themselves. If I could get this drug, I would have to inject myself too. I would have to beat a lifelong fear. This all would be fine if I lived just one mile away from where I live now because one mile away is the Bath and North East Somerset (B&NES) Health Authority. B&NES offers the drug Beta Interferon on the National Health Service but in Wiltshire, where I lived, the Health Authority deemed it as far too expensive. I wonder what difference that one mile really makes. Why should one mile be the difference between life and death? The difference between me being offered a chance to live my teenage life in the way that all the other teenagers did or the other option of not getting the drug, to continue deteriorating until my eyesight was null and my walking was impossible, until the shine in my eyes turned to sheer depression and to a life I no longer wanted to live. What? I thought this was a National Health Service? How can you not prescribe a drug just because of the county you live in? Surreal, I thought. A nightmare that should never ever happen.

'Stephanie, you will have to make a choice.' My mum's voice strong and determined. 'Would you like to stay quiet and ignore the illness, to not get the drug, or would you like to go public, show the whole country that you have MS and that you need the drug?'

I decided to do the latter option. I contacted the local newspaper telling them how appalled I was that a seventeen year old child couldn't get the drug they needed because of where they lived. Lots of newspapers contacted me and I was publicised in some way every day, my picture almost being the face of MS, the fight for equal opportunities.

My local MP, James Gray, was a real support, insisting I go to the House of Commons while he fought my case in front of the then-Prime Minister, Tony Blair. My dad wrote many letters asking for anyone's help. Meanwhile, I was getting sicker and the depression I was trying to fight was ever-increasing. Why was I bothering to fight anyway? I was finished, my dreams had died, my life was over. Why was I fighting to learn how to inject myself? My life was a dismal mess and the strength by my side was my mum, strong and proud, trying always to take my pain away. She said to me once 'I wish I had the MS. I have lived my life already, yours is just beginning.' This made me cry then and it still does now. She wanted to take my pain away, to put herself in the way of an oncoming truck so she got hurt and I was saved. I thought this was the nicest thing to say and I believe if it was possible to take the illness off me she would be the first to take it.

I grew stronger after she said this because if she wants to take my illness away she obviously wants me in her life; she wants me to keep going. If I never find a husband or if I get very sick, my mum will be there for me. She will dry my tears, she will be the rock by my side. I need to get this drug to help me and to keep my mum strong, to stop her worrying about me. This fight is no longer just about me; it is for the whole family. I need to get the drug, get better and then I won't be such a problem. I have to give everyone the chance to get over my illness and to move on with their own lives irrelevant of whether I am sick or well. I need to grow up and get over my broken childhood. I have to be an adult and I have to get stronger. I can't give up yet. I have a drug and a new life to fight for.

CHAPTER 24

Letters – Stephanie to Tony Blair

Mike & Linda Millward
Box, Corsham
Wiltshire,

1 March 2000

Dear Mr Blair,

I realise that you must have many requests. What makes this one different is that it's a request for help for an England Swimming International. Our daughter, Stephanie, is 18 years old. She was expecting to be battling to go to Sydney 2000; now she is battling Multiple Sclerosis (MS).

Stephanie was the English Schools Champion & record holder, as well as the National Age Group Champion and record holder at backstroke. She trained with the Olympic swimmers at Bath University & represented England as a full international at the 1998 World Cup meetings.

Stephanie first demonstrated problems with her balance in March 1999, shortly after returning from China for the World

Schools Games. We believe that the inoculations she received for the trip may be linked to her illness. Further research is required before the link between immunisation for hepatitis and MS can be clearly established.

Stephanie is a lovely looking girl, more like a model than the stereo-type swimmer. As a swimmer her strength was in her beauty and grace within the water - even people who had no real knowledge of swimming stated on many occasions that they could just watch her all day. Now she has stopped swimming completely, is unsteady on her feet, has difficulty concentrating and is finding her A-level examinations very difficult. Her neurologist, Dr Dawson, is worried about her progressive deterioration. She is currently undergoing intravenous steroid treatment but this is just a holding treatment. What she needs is the opportunity to receive Beta Interferon which is currently the only drug which has an effect against this terrible disease. We live in a postcode area, Wiltshire, (Stephanie was the 1998 Wiltshire Sports personality) which doesn't support Beta Interferon.

We have always supported Stephanie and our three other children, and we all continue to support her in her fight against MS. Mr James Gray MP for Wiltshire has invited Stephanie to visit the House of Commons on 8 March as part of the MS Action Day campaign. We are eagerly awaiting the decision of the National Institute of Clinical Excellence (NICE) committee as to whether Beta Interferon will be funded. What happens if the answer is no? While we would be willing to contribute to the yearly cost of £10,000 we cannot fund it completely. Is there anything you can do to help us?

Stephanie gave a lot in her quest to be the best, both for herself and for her desire to represent England. Is there anything that can be done in return to help her? Stephanie is a wonderful opportunity to promote any number of initiatives. We are not requesting charity, only help and hope.

Yours sincerely,
Mike & Linda Millward

cc:Alan Milburn MP Secretary of State for Health.
James Gray MP
Dr Dawson – Royal United Hospital, Bath
Wiltshire Health Authority.
Schering Health Care Ltd.

CHAPTER 25

House of Commons

My fight just kept on going: were they ever going to give in and let me have the drug? It was obvious that I should be allowed to have the drug as it is supposed to be a National Health Service. My parents have paid a lot of taxes towards the NHS so why, therefore, when I need their help is it not allowed? Surely I should be offered a fair chance, the ability to try to get better.

The strong media attention in my case made me feel stronger and made me feel that I deserved the chance to try the drug Beta Interferon in case it helped me. I was seventeen years old, a baby really, and I didn't want the illness, the disease, to ruin my life at this early age. My local MP, Mr James Gray, approached me and asked if I would like his help. I obviously said yes and on the required day I was driven up to the House of Commons in a limo with James Gray and my parents. When the taxi stopped and the door was opened for me I got out to the sound of hundreds of cameras. My bright red skirt suit made me look the picture of health. My parents got out of the taxi too and we followed James Gray before I was stopped for photos and many questions. I was all smiles and answered every question with determination and desire allowing the papers the right to believe that I had a chance to turn the Health Authorities around, to make them bend over backwards to help me. I knew I looked like a film star with my long blonde hair and blue-green eyes.

The red suit just made me stand out, the person in the centre of the picture. I loved all the attention and I felt as though I had reached all the goals I had previously aimed to get: the Olympic gold; the records. I felt that I was holding every MS sufferer's hand and telling them that I was given MS to help them, to get rid of the unfairness in the country.

I was very confident as I followed James Gray into the parliament buildings. The crowds stayed outside and I noted the picturesque building with all the stone work and pictures; it was all stunning. I walked through with a smile on my face knowing that this was where I was meant to be. I took a seat next to my mum in the main room and watched all the opening ceremonies as the MPs walked in. My parents and I watched as the MPs discussed other issues and when James Gray stood up I got excited - this was my bit! James Gray talked about one of his constituents (me) and how it was unfair that I hadn't been offered the drug. The other MPs listened and agreed that I should be allowed the drug at least to see if it works. I wish it had been their choice but obviously life isn't that easy.

When the meeting was over I walked out uncertain if it had been a positive meeting or even whether anything had been decided. The media jumped on me again when I walked out of the House of Commons and again I smiled and answered the questions hoping that this was all going to work in my favour. James Gray took us for cup of tea and agreed that it had been a good meeting and that hopefully something good would happen.

The following day my face graced the front of all the national and local papers and the red suit looked the perfect choice. Yes, everything was going well. Maybe I will get the drug!!

Stephanie Millward – the face of MS.

CHAPTER 26

Letters – Stephanie to Wiltshire Health

Mike Millward
Box
Corsham
Wiltshire

28 March 2000

Ref: Stephanie Millward
Ref: Millward02b - Jeremy Hallett Chief Executive Wiltshire Health
Authority

To: Dr Dawson, Royal United Hospital NHS Trust

Dear Dr Dawson,

With specific reference to the letter I received from Mr Hallett
dated 16 March 2000 in which he offered the use of the Wiltshire
Health Authority appeal process, I would like to take the opportunity of lodging an appeal on behalf of Stephanie through this
process with Prof. Philip Milner Director of Public Health WHA.

While I realise that you will be providing details on Stephanie from a clinical perspective, I would like to also offer the following justification which I believe are also worthy of consideration, if not already part of your clinical observations.

Stephanie is only 18 years of age. This is a very young age at which to be diagnosed with Multiple Sclerosis. Because she is so young Stephanie should be offered the opportunity to regain a full life for as long as possible.

Stephanie, we believe, is a suitable candidate for Beta Interferon and she has only recently been diagnosed. Beta Interferon is most effective on newly-diagnosed, young people.

The benefit of Beta Interferon is effective only for certain people. Surely the cost of determining its success on Stephanie is worth the £10,000 per year to find out. If it is successful then the cost is one that can be justified as it produces results, if it isn't beneficial then the cost is minimised as it will only apply for the period she takes the treatment.

Stephanie being treated, or not, must be done in a comparable manner no matter where she lives. Why is it that she does not even have the option of the drug in Wiltshire but would in other Health Authorities? This is inconsistent and unfair. I feel this is a form of discrimination. We, as a country, are trying to fight against discrimination in its many guises; isn't this just another example that the current policy of WHA is condoning?

It also appears to me a strong financial case is realised by Wiltshire County Council, and I suspect the National Health Service as a whole by financial planning on a long-term basis. Initial spending to eliminate or reduce the overall whole life cost of the problem surely makes sense?

Government Health initiatives are focused upon prevention rather than cure. Surely provision of a treatment to prevent further deterioration follows this direction.

The financial cost of supporting a MS patient is high. I believe these costs are far higher than the yearly £10,000 spent delaying the full impact of MS and allowing the sufferer to lead a more normal life, contributing to the community.

The latest indications given by the MS Society Chief Medical Officer in a recent lecture was that, in his opinion, the cause (shortly followed by the cure) of MS now has a medium term prognosis, circa 5 years. Stephanie should be given the opportunity to take advantage of this expected breakthrough.

The moral justification in supporting a member of the community who has shown dedication and commitment in pursuing a sporting goal ultimately with the aim of winning a medal at the Olympics.

As an athlete, Stephanie demonstrated a constant awareness of what she could eat and she has continued with this commitment following a very strict low-fat diet in an attempt to combat MS. This commitment should be taken advantage of. Stephanie has never taken recreational drugs, smoked and has only recently taken any form of alcohol. Stephanie hadn't ever visited the doctor for any health problems before her illness. This demonstrates a basically fit and well individual on which to begin combating MS as well as one that hadn't previously been a cost to the Health Service. There are no other cases of Multiple Sclerosis or similar within our family.

To summarise, our position with Stephanie is one of looking for equal opportunity and hope.

I appreciate your constraints on this issue but also hope that our position is understandable and suggestions worthy of consideration by yourself and Wiltshire Health Authority.

Yours sincerely,
Mike Millward

c.c. Jeremy Hallett – Chief Executive Wilts Health Authority
James Gray MP
Prof. Philip Milner Director of Public Health WHA

CHAPTER 27
Dear David Gledhill

(To the editor of *Bath Chronicle* Newspaper)

Dear David,

This is just a little note to say THANK YOU for your help in getting me the drug to fight my MS. I cannot begin to tell you how much you have helped me over these past few months, physically and mentally. Without your help, I would still be struggling to come to terms with the disease, but your continuous support has shown me that there are people around me who really want to help.

I think that you and the whole *Bath Chronicle* crew, deserve a GOLD medal for the support that you have so kindly given to me.

I believe that it was your support, along with the loving support of my family, that turned me from being a depressed and very ill little girl to being a happy, strong, inspirational young woman who is now so full-of-life. I have started swimming again, once a week. How far will I get now?

I am also trying hard at school, especially as I am currently taking my A-level exams, whereas before I met you and David West, I had given up on all my school work.

All I have left to say is THANK YOU. THANK YOU for everything that you have done for me. THANK YOU so much for helping me to get the life-enhancing drug that will hopefully return me to being the happy, promising, perfectly able young girl that I was before I came into contact with my debilitating disease.

I will never be able to thank you enough but if you ever need anyone to go and watch a show at the Theatre Royal again, I would definitely help you out!

Thanks again.

All my love,
Stephanie Millward

CHAPTER 28

Hearts of Pure Gold

We eventually won the fight and I was awarded the drug on a trial basis until NICE decided whether it was cost effective enough or not. We also won it for a number of other MS sufferers, although each one had to meet the specific criteria stated. A number of MS 'friends' didn't meet the criteria and so were not awarded it and their reaction was to turn against me which was a shame.

I have so many people I wish to thank for all the ways that they helped me during this particularly hard period in my life. The main ones obviously being my mum who has a heart of pure gold and Adrian McHugh, who will enter my life later in this book. I also met a nice young man called David West who went out of his way to raise the profile of my case to get the drug Betaferon. David contacted everybody he could think of, and promoted me in every way possible; he was fantastic. David had this way that just made everyone give him donations and they offered everything to try to help in some way. It was amazing and I watched in wonder as David went to everyone trying to fund the £12,000 for my year's supply of Beta Interferon when the Health Authority originally said that I was not worthy!

Another guy I need to thank is the well-known actor, Clive Mantle (who played a doctor in 'Casualty'), lives close to my home in Box, Wiltshire, who also tried everything to promote my story. He was on the radio being interviewed about me all the time and I was lucky enough to stand right next to him as the newspapers took loads of photos. Clive Mantle is one of my heroes!

I need to thank a good friend of mine, Paul Langely, the owner of the Manor Garage in Box who also helped me in many ways. Firstly, he saw my poem 'Paying the Price' in the local paper and he spoke to his friends to get singers and musicians to play this poem as a song to raise money for the possible Nerve Centre to be built at Frenchay Hospital, Bristol, which was initially meant to be an MS centre. There wasn't much help for MS sufferers in the areas around where I lived but a guy called John decided he wanted to change a stable block behind Bristol's Frenchay hospital in to an MS centre (the MS Nerve Centre). John started fundraising for the £1.5 million needed and when he had received almost the whole amount from loving donations he was forced to give every penny back as the plans for the building fell through. What a shame, was my thought as I had also been part of his fundraising team. I feel that all the people who helped me had hearts of gold to try anything and everything to raise the money for either me or for the Nerve Centre. I could not have done it without their graciousness. Paul Langely also helped me to walk across the road from the Manor Garage to the Co-operative store when I worked there. This was fantastic as my legs often proved difficult and all the help he gave me was fantastic! Paul literally stopped the traffic so I could walk across without any problem! An amazing man!

The media grabbed my story with open arms and I definitely became the face of MS. GMTV interviewed me and my dad on one occasion and I still hold a copy of this, although watching it makes me shy away as I hear my slurred and very slow words and watch as I struggle to smile and fight against the illness. It makes me feel proud that GMTV wanted to help me fight to get the drug. I also have lots of newspaper clippings of my fight for the drug which makes me smile because of the huge support that I received from Wiltshire, my home county, and that wonderful newspaper, the *Bath Chronicle*.

After six months of campaigning I was awarded the drug Betaferon on a trial basis under the NHS. This meant that I was given the drug for free and it was paid for by Wiltshire's Health Authority who had said originally they would not fund it. I was delighted about this and started on the drug as soon as I could. I believe that because I was allowed the drug a number of other individuals in Wiltshire and other postcode lottery areas were also allowed it. This was therefore a massive benefit for anybody involved and a relief for a number of MS sufferers who deemed their lives unworthy of hope.

It is nice to know that whenever you need somebody's help they will almost bend over backwards to help you. There really are people alive with hearts of pure GOLD.

CHAPTER 29

Needles

Betaferon B is meant to be my lifeline, a form of medication that will help me get my legs and therefore my life back again. The only problem I had was the fact that I would have to inject myself every other day for the rest of my life which, to me, seemed like a horror story. I had always had a fear of needles, remembering all too clearly going to the doctors in Saudi Arabia and hiding under the doctor's table. Again, just before the World Cup competition in Shanghai, when I was sick with a cold, a sore throat and ear ache and I still had to have the injection which, in my opinion, will always be my probable cause of MS. Now I had to inject myself. A nightmare. A horror story come true.

While life was going on as normal outside I sat on my bed with an empty syringe and a needle in my hands. Picking up the vial and vial adapter I insert the adapter into the vial then the syringe into the adapter, pushing down and releasing the liquid into the powder. I turned the vial to mix the products and pulled back tapping out any bubbles. Finally, I took the syringe out of the adapter and pushed the needle to the top of the syringe. With the injection all prepared I dreaded what was coming next.

My anticipation of me trying to push it in again, a reminder that I am not normal. I then think to myself, did I do it yesterday? If I did it yesterday I don't have to do it today! But no, I know I didn't. The needles feel like they come around every day and they come around so fast each, one reminding me it will be there again soon. Did I do it today? No, so therefore it is tomorrow. One day off but all day thinking, tomorrow I will have to inject again. Tomorrow which comes so fast and it is injection time again. The tomorrow, the rest day that never seems to come.

Maybe if I inject two or three times a day every day, maybe this will rid me of this disease? Maybe if I overdose on Betaferon I will be back to normal, all better again, and I could go and swim the races I was dragged away from. Maybe hundreds of needles will rid me of MS, maybe I can have my Olympic dreams back again.

No, reality bites as the needle touches my pinched stomach, the prick causing me to close my eyes and a tear to drain from my eyes. The needle pressed into my stomach, a soft area and nicer than the leg as it hurts too much there. The stomach always seems to be the easiest place to inject. Mental strength pushes it in; it hurts and the tears that nobody ever sees or hears fall. I switch the light off as this is the best thing for me to do after an injection. My own world with aches and pains and my own solemn life with the needles and the pain. Flu-like symptoms will be my reaction to the needles and I try to fall asleep so that I don't feel any of it. Fall asleep, then tomorrow I am free but still with the knowledge that the next day I will have to inject again. What a dismal end to all my naïve Olympic dreams. What a miserable existence. What horrendous thing did I do to deserve this horrible life?

CHAPTER 30

10 Downing Street

Dear Stephanie,

As part of the Multiple Sclerosis Society, I would like to invite you to 10 Downing Street to meet Cherie Blair.

Wow! I get to go to 10 Downing Street! The invitation was sent from the MS Society who had been invited to go to 10 Downing Street and they had decided I was the perfect person to go.

My dad met me in London when I walked out of the Underground station. We walked down the road chatting merrily about where I was going and what I was going to say. I was very excited as I had seen the outside of this house many times on the TV and had wondered what the rooms inside would look like and how posh it all would be. Here was my chance to find out!

'Hi ya!' Paul was walking towards us. Paul worked in London so it was easy for him to come over to meet us.

'Hi Paul!' I replied.

We walked together up towards the main entrance where I walked through the security gates leaving Dad and Paul on the main road waiting for me to return. I had to put my bag through the machine to be checked. I then had to walk through the security detector which thankfully did not beep.

I went to the front door and it looked, not surprisingly, the same as it does on the TV.

I went inside and the first thing I noticed was how expensive the ceiling looked. What a waste of tax payers' money I thought. I am sure white paint would have been just fine. The hallway was quite small and the rooms weren't nearly as large as I had anticipated. If I was Prime Minister I am sure I would extend the house and make it look far more exciting. The only good part was the ceiling and who looks up? Well, apart from me!

I went upstairs as directed and stood in the queue waiting to be introduced to Cherie Blair. I felt a little like I was standing in a queue to see the dentist. I was scared but excited. Also in the line were the very famous Alistair Hignell and his wife, Jeannie, along with a few other individuals, probably from the MS Society. Alastair Hignell had just retired as a rugby player for Bath and was also an Ex England international player! An amazing person! My turn came and I felt quite worried. What if she hated me? Cherie was a lot smaller than I had anticipated and with my heels I felt very tall in comparison! She was very kind when I was introduced to her by one of the guys from the MS Society. She wished me good luck for my life and my swimming. I didn't tell her that my swimming career was over and that this was a sore subject for me. I decided I liked her but was annoyed that Tony, her husband, had been forced to go to Israel as opposed to meeting me!

I moved forward and was handed a glass of wine. This was probably a bad idea I decided because I was feeling pretty tired anyway. I went over to Alastair and started chatting. I found both him and Jeanie very comforting and interesting people and I asked for their phone number which they gave me straight away. I started sipping the wine feeling very young in the crowd. The wine is bound to make me look older, I thought.

Cherie stood at the front and started talking about how nice it was to meet us. Generally, I hate these speeches because they have all been written beforehand and are not straight from the heart and therefore often tediously boring. She then invited one of the MS Society's speakers to say a few words. I decided to sit down on one of the sofas in the room; the fatigue caused by my MS was exhausting me.

Just shut my eyes for one minute...

Open. I will look stupid if I fall asleep here. It is a bit boring, maybe just a minute...

I had fallen asleep on the coach and when I was woken a few minutes later I must have gone very red with the embarrassment! Well at least I can say I am probably the only visitor who has ever fallen asleep when visiting 10 Downing Street!

A couple of hours later after lots of polite chatting and a few white wines, I went outside into the cold night and saw my brother and dad with quizzical looks on their faces. I smiled to say it had been good and they smiled back. I had to go back through security before I was allowed back onto the main road.

'It was really good,' I said with a huge smile on my face. 'But they have spent a lot of tax payer s' money on little things that I am sure they don't need.' Always straight to the point!

Well, that was an experience I will never forget and probably one I wouldn't have got without the MS, so thank you, MS!

CHAPTER 31

MS - My War

An incurable illness, no cure no treatment
A debilitating disease – a fight, my war
Why does my life hurt me so much?
When will all the pain be gone?

I am a survivor, but I want to die
I am a fighter but I want to quit
A large battle that I am now losing
An endless war, I cannot win.

Look in the mirror see a smile on your face
Look inside see a life full of pain
MS is invisible, I can disguise my health
MS destroys lives, can't hide from myself.

I try to look up but my life is declining
I stare at the stars but my life is still sliding
Who's going to help me rid my life of the pain?
Who can I rely on to relight my life flame?

We are waiting for a life
But will a cure ever be found?
My heart has been broken, leaving two halves
The cure, my lifesaver, will rebind my heart.

I will then be able to realise my dreams
The future fears will all be gone
The pain will be tied down and controlled
The torturing disease locked up behind bars.

MS breaks a thousand hearts
Heart and feelings, Hopes and dreams
The cure will end my life of worries
When will that special second ever be?

I am a survivor, I can't fade away
I am a fighter so I will not give in
A large battle that I will not lose
An endless war, I have to win.

Stephanie Millward Copyright 2000

CHAPTER 32

Paul

Paul, my big brother. What can I say? Grown up well before his time. At the age of four he was as mature as a ten-year-old. By eighteen his sub-conscious had planned for him to be a multi-millionaire and he had planned on moving away and travelling the world. Paul is like a rock; strong and never faltering. He is one of the most determined people I know and I expect he always will be a strength by my side. He is my big brother, strong and almost a hero in my eyes. If I need any help he is always there for me.

On one occasion, when we were out drinking and dancing, my MS got the better of me and so Paul slung one of my arms around his shoulder and practically dragged me to the taxi rank where he pushed in the front, got me into the taxi and then paid the taxi driver extra to make sure he helped me to my front door. The taxi driver did exactly what he had been told to do and I was helped to the door before the concerned driver drove away. Paul had made sure I was safe before he had even thought about enjoying his own evening.

Paul is often very quiet, living inside his head. He seems to size up any person that he has just met before asking relevant questions about that person. Paul has never been interested in fashion and was once even seen wearing a top belonging to one of Nicholas's girl-friends! Thankfully, Kristy is very fashion conscious and keeps him in check. Paul also drove a little Metro even when he was working in

London earning a small fortune but then gave this car to Nicholas, to help with his driving lessons, before buying a second hand Audi A3 which he later gave to my mum, which she loves!

Once, when he was in the UK, I went swimming with Paul in the Springfield centre in Corsham. I had a set of 20x100m Freestyle to swim and Paul swam them all with me even though he was not fit, and then, for the last 2x100m, he asked me to race him, so I did. We both swam a 1 minute and twelve seconds and burst out laughing before setting off again after only ten seconds' rest! Paul has all this determination, I am sure he would have been an Olympic champion if he hadn't been so busy organising and contemplating his million-aire plans.

I find myself looking up to Paul, believing that I can be like him when I am older; I want to be strong, I want to be self-assured. I feel very lucky that I was next in my family line: Paul, bright and perfect; me, blonde, blue eyes; Kristy, brilliant in every way; Mister the brains who fights to be on the top of a pretty big pile of success stories! Paul led us all out and showed us the way forward, putting stars in our eyes and even helping to bring our dreams closer. I firmly believe that I am privileged to have Paul as my big brother.

CHAPTER 33
Sydney, Australia

Dripping water, running down my neck. I had put all my Beta Interferon needles in a box above my head and it was full of ice that was obviously melting. The cold chill reminded me of the needles being pushed into me. A reminder that I am sick. The twenty-four hours travelling seemed to last forever and my friend, Leanne, and I spent the majority of the time watching films or sleeping. Thankfully there were no kids screaming or running up and down the aisles. Thankfully I could sit and think about life and all of its possibilities. I was flying to Sydney, the same place that the Olympic Games had been held many months before, the same Games I should have been swimming in. I could go and visit the main sites or see the pool I would have swam in. I had pictured coming here to swim at the Olympics in the year 2000 but the circumstances were so incredibly different now.

My parents had wanted to help me by buying me tickets to go see my brother Paul who was now living and working in Sydney, Australia. Leanne had also wanted to visit Australia and said she would come with me. We had been so excited about seeing all the sites, such as the Opera house, and enjoying the sun and the heat; we had been discussing everything we had wanted to see. We were very excited when we packed our bags and even more so when we arrived at the airport ready for our flight. The flight was supposed to take the full twenty-four hours with one fuelling stop after twenty hours of flying. I loved flying so the length of time didn't worry me at all and it was only when the ice was dripping on my neck and the airplane was too cold and the films were boring that I realised how long twenty-four hours actually was.

Paul met us at the airport and helped collect our bags before we got into a taxi. Paul lived on Manly Island, so we had to catch a boat to go over to the island and then had to walk to Paul's flat. Unfortunately, Paul had chosen a flat which was situated almost at the top of a hill and dragging suitcases up this hill was harder than anticipated! We unpacked our bags and rested with a big cup of tea before we started chatting about the things we could and would do. See the sights in Australia! See the Sydney Opera house! Go shopping in Sydney! See the Sydney Harbour Bridge! Hopefully see some koalas! Australia was a whole new world and I expected it to be a wonderful adventure for us.

Paul introduced Leanne and me to his friends and told us how to get everywhere. The next day Paul had to go to work so Leanne and I decided to hit the shops. To get to the shops we had to catch the boat to get to the mainland and then had to walk a short distance to catch another boat that took us to the main part of Sydney. This was all very exciting. We paid the money and jumped aboard seeing the sights and hearing the sounds of Manly Island. What a great way to get to Sydney and how exciting! Unfortunately almost straight away I struggled to walk any distance. I was very angry that I could not be the same as any other tourist. My MS was completely in charge on this trip but Leanne was very patient with me. We had to endure many breaks while my legs decided whether or not they were going to move. I kept the optimistic smile on my face with the desire inside to just break down and cry. Keep moving legs keep going, but no. They eventually stopped fully and we had to call the taxi to help us.

When we got back to Paul's flat I realised something else very important: I had left the vial adaptors at home. The vial adaptors help to make up the injection. This meant that I couldn't have an injection while in Sydney. What a stupid mistake to make. How depressing. In the end my mum organised to fly the injection parts over for me. I can breathe again! The parts were sent and everything was sorted but I still struggled with walking and we spent so much time resting that we didn't get around to seeing any of the sights we had originally planned to see. Sydney will always be a place of unease for me personally. Nothing good has happened for me there. I wish it had all be different. While in Australia it rained often and a nasty car driver hit a puddle covering me and Leanne in dirty water. I was furious but there was nothing we could do about it.

I was so stressed with the MS being in charge and me and my good friend just trying to cope with the disasters every day that we were soon wishing the time away and only wanted to go home. I told my mum that we had had enough and that the MS was winning this fight. My mum in her loving way arranged for her home insurance to pay for me to come home early. I was crying non-stop and I felt like such a failure and such a mistake. I had let Leanne, my mum and Paul down as well as myself. I felt like a miserable failure. I was so useless.

CHAPTER 34
Confused and Frustrated

I was annoyed, angry and upset, fed up with everything that life had to offer. It just didn't make sense. I was not able to understand anything and everything seemed to confuse me. Life was so hard and everything was becoming a fight. I got bitter about uncontrollable things, such as the traffic which made me very angry when there was absolutely nothing I could have done about it. Everything annoyed me so much. I just felt I had let myself down again, that I wasn't good enough.

On one occasion I was driving to a venue and I was late because of the traffic, but being late didn't affect anyone else, and it is something that I really should be able to control. It is something that happens often, and really isn't that important but I was furious, screaming and shouting at the 'bad' drivers from inside my car. Everything just annoyed me so much. Everything seemed to confuse me and I got annoyed about everything that happened.

I had to learn to drive with MS and pass my driving test with MS. When I went to take my first driving test I had to say straight away to the examiner, 'I have MS'. The driving examiner obviously thought FAIL, FAIL, FAIL, and I did. I then started driving an automatic car to help with the trouble I was having with my left leg. It was so much easier and thankfully I passed my test the second time.

When the examiner said, 'Pass', I asked, 'Really?', not believing it.

'Yeah, you drove well. You have passed.'

'Even with the MS?'

'Yeah, I feel you are safe enough to drive even with your MS.'

Wow I never expected that! Everybody learns to drive and passes almost straight away but I didn't deserve to pass. I have MS. The pass was like a huge 'congratulations' for me and it gave me confidence that maybe my life wasn't as bad as I first thought. I can drive now! The MS hasn't got in the way of that one!

Anger, my uncontrollable anger. The anger was almost expected as my doctor pre-warned it as part of grieving. But anger all the time? Why does everybody seem to have such easy lives? What did I do wrong?

I paid to do an A-level exam to make myself a cleverer, better person but my memory just didn't remember anything. I spent days repeating the page over and over again until I could almost read it out loud but then I tried to move to my next page and the whole of the first page had been forgotten. All the work I had done had completely disappeared. I used to be an extremely clever and bright person who now had this ill brain that kept forgetting things; I felt I had let myself down again. How did I get sick? I ate all the right things and did everything perfectly. Where the hell did I go so wrong?

This illness had attacked the memory part of my brain. The part that was needed to remember my past and to remember everything important. I felt as though everything had been lost: my wonderful memories; the life I was told to grieve for; the person I so wanted to be again.

Who is in control of our lives or our life paths?

Is the devil playing a game with my mind and with my heart and soul? Is he in control of all this pain I feel and is he in control of inevitably what will become of me?

But there is a God up there too, why isn't he fighting for me? Did I really do something that bad?

Maybe they are both trying to teach me a lesson? Maybe they are trying to make me stronger and make me do something important. Maybe these hard parts are just lessons trying to make sure that everything I do is for the good of mankind, myself or of someone else. Maybe I am meant to become someone that people look up to. Maybe I am going to become a hero for someone else. I love helping people and I love helping to enable people to smile. Maybe my pain will lead to strength which will lead to courage and an undying positivity. Maybe my fight is going to help others become something they had barely even dreamed about. Maybe I will be able to help people turn their lives around for the better. Maybe both God and the devil are teaching me important lessons, the lessons that no one will ever be able to pay for.

Being in a state of confusion and frustration is really annoying but it must be a good thing as it is making me stronger as a person! I often have to ask people only to say one question at a time or to speak a bit slower so that all of the information goes into my brain and is then organised so that I can prepare to reply.

These lessons are making me stronger and better as a person! I can learn to live with MS; all I need is to be in control. I need to learn how to live with it all, to understand what makes it happy and what makes it angry. I need to learn how to be in charge of the MS almost as if it was a child. What things will make it cry and what things, therefore will, make it smile? MS can and will eventually end my life so I need to make sure that I am the stronger one.

I need to win this endless war. I must be the winner.

CHAPTER 35

Anger Management

'Stephanie, you need to raise your self-esteem. The MS has taken the dream but just remember all the wonderful things you did before you got sick.' Mums always know best even when their child is fighting for life. I listened to my her words and decided that I did have to do something as I had spent almost eight years now doing nothing but grieving, working and crying.

I went to my doctor to discuss self-esteem and she said that the first thing I had to do was to go on an anger management course. Anger management? Why do I have to go on an anger management course? I'm not angry. Am I?

The doctor convinced me, and, walking into the first session at Chippenham Hospital, I felt worried. I was sure there would be just the angry teenagers who weren't doing well at school or druggies who couldn't control their temper but I was pleasantly surprised. The room was full of many people of different age groups and both women and men were there. I sat down on my own but was quickly joined by three pleasant ladies who said 'Good morning' with a nice smile on their faces. I felt better because of this and felt more confident that my preconceptions were not realised on this occasion.

The tutor of the course told us a story about two young girls who were brought up in entirely different houses. One was told to have breakfast before school and then catch the bus at 8am. The second had to wake up early to walk her family's two dogs and to feed her sister and take her sister to nursery before walking to school herself. The second had to eat breakfast at school which annoyed the first as she thought she should get up earlier to have her breakfast before school. The first was annoyed by the second until she asked why was she eating in class, and found out the reason was that she has so many jobs to do in the morning before school. People judge others by the things they see. This course taught me to look further than the face as each person has a truly different story to tell.

The course helped me to see why other people often annoy me and made me realise that life is generally just a series of coincidences adjusted or changed by your own decisions. I had always felt that the more you tried to do things well the better your outcomes should be and therefore that the kinder you treat others the nicer the things that will happen to you. When I got MS I realised that things don't happen to you because of something you did before. I learnt in science that every action equals an equal and opposite reaction, so therefore in my case every action does not necessarily equal an equal and opposite reaction, and that not every good thing I have done in my life will necessarily deserve a beneficial or positive reaction in return.

I feel privileged to have gone on this course and believe that this has helped me with people in general. I can now relate to just about everyone and can feel at ease with rebellious or very angry people. I just have to trust that it was the way they were brought up and that the people they have met in their lives have shaped them into who they are now and that they are not just nasty people. Everybody has an open book that they will write with the decisions that they chose.

Good luck to everyone. I hope you make all the right decisions or at least decisions that will end up teaching you brilliant lessons!

CHAPTER 36
Mum's Version

The nightmare started on 7 May 1999 when Stephanie began to feel unwell. The GP assured us that there was no cause for concern but decided to refer her to an ENT specialist at the local hospital believing her symptoms of dizziness and vertigo may have been due to an inner ear infection. While doing an examination the ENT specialist noticed unusual, rapid movements in her pupils and called in his colleague, a neurological consultant. The neurologist, who turned out to be Dr Ken Dawson invited Stephanie back for more neurological examinations. Stephanie was later sent for a MRI scan; believing that not much was wrong with her, she smiled through it. At this point Stephanie could not have looked more beautiful or fit.

We decided to go privately so that we could find out quickly what was wrong with Stephanie as she wanted to get back into the water to train for her next competition. The results of the scan were due in two days' time. Stephanie carried on training. During the next day's training session the coach called me to collect Stephanie as she couldn't read the clock and kept on bumping into the other swimmers - she was also very shaky and wobbly when she got out of the pool. We were not to know it then but this would be the last time that Stephanie swam in the Bath University pool and signal the end of her life as a swimmer.

Stephanie's results were due the following day; her driving test was also scheduled. The instructor decided that due to Stephanie's dizziness it would be better to cancel the test which we duly did. This was just the beginning of many such cancellations. Waiting for the results during that day was a nightmare; my mind was on overdrive imagining all kinds of illnesses, most specifically a brain tumour.

The appointment was a very slow process in which Dr Dawson examined Stephanie thoroughly first and the, much later, told us the results of the MRI scan. He told us that he had found widespread lesions on her brain which could be due to a recent virus or possibly Multiple Sclerosis. He was hoping that it was the former and that Stephanie's symptoms would disappear and there would be no need for further action or appointments. Unfortunately it was to be the latter.

We knew nothing of MS, and the doctor told us not to read any books on the subject and to just forget the possibility. Stephanie seemed fine - she was seventeen and at that point in her life always expecting her glass to be half-full, not half-empty. In other words, she was extremely positive. She seemed relieved that it was not a tumour. The doctor asked us what we thought it would be - my answer was the tumour and Mike's was Mad Cow's Disease. Dr Dawson told Stephanie to carry on with her life as normal and to do as much as she felt able. She was even planning to be back training for the National Championships which would take place in July. For me, treating Stephanie as normal with swellings on the brain was impossible. I wanted to wrap her up in cotton wool. I felt useless and that there was nothing I could do for her to make her better.

Stephanie would not allow herself to be sick and have time off school - she carried on as usual, apart from swimming. This period of time, although worrying, was probably the easiest time of the illness as Stephanie was still very positive. She still felt the whole thing would just go away and that there was every chance she would go back to her former life and continuous training.

I did buy and read books on MS which absolutely terrified me. I read them in private. I didn't want her to worry about the possibility of her having this chronic, debilitating disease at seventeen years old.

The days turned into weeks and Stephanie's condition did not improve, in fact it deteriorated. Her sleep pattern became very erratic and more symptoms appeared. Her memory became impaired and she found it very difficult to retain any information she had learned during her A-level lessons. I became more worried about Stephanie as she became depressed and irritable because she was unable to swim. She was also getting very worried about not being able to retain information; she understood during the lessons but as soon as the lesson had finished the information disappeared from her memory. She started to panic as she had been above average and had always found her studies easy; this was a new experience for Stephanie. Because she had always found school easy she had been able to carry on with training and do A-levels simultaneously.

Stephanie read about and started a new low-fat diet with high poly-unsaturates and almost no saturated fat. She excluded many things from her diet including chocolate, ice cream, crisps, red meat etc. She starting taking large amounts of primrose oil capsules, vitamins and minerals as described in an MS book. This new diet seemed to alleviate some of her symptoms.

The whole family went on holiday to Tenerife which Stephanie enjoyed, apart from falling a few times and having feelings of tiredness. She seemed well on this holiday. She also went to Spain with her boyfriend and his family for a week which was not as successful - she went horse riding and realised that this was another thing that she could no longer do. She could not get on the horse as her legs were too weak. During this holiday more symptoms appeared such as her right leg giving way.

Also, during this time she had no periods whatsoever, so the doctor sent her for a scan which turned out to be normal. She had to wait many more months for her periods to return to normal. Stephanie was also becoming more and more frustrated that she could not go to Bath University training. However, she returned to Corsham Swimming Club but felt that she was becoming slow so did not enjoy it. She also had extremely bad symptoms and was unable to walk back to the changing rooms after a training session. I saw her once during one of these sessions and I was so upset I could not go back with her to watch her swim. It was as though she was already crippled and the beautiful, graceful and coordinated movements that enabled Stephanie to swim so fast previously had disappeared. It was a nightmare.

Stephanie still tried to run and train but it was almost impossible. She had previously bought a treadmill from funds that she had won when she was voted Junior North Wilts Sports Personality of the Year, and she tried to use this daily. At this point her legs were still working when she wanted them to, but she was only able to run for approximately 5 minutes when previously she would run for at least a half an hour. She was very stressed knowing that she was losing all the fitness she had worked so hard to build up.

On her return from holiday she went to collect the results of her maths module which she had failed. Stephanie was extremely upset about this as maths was always one of Stephanie's strong points. She decided then that she would drop maths and carry on with her other two A-levels in economics and biology. This was just the start of Stephanie trying to come to terms with failure, as she had not known it before.

Just after a Christmas when Stephanie's symptoms worsened slightly we went again to see Dr Dawson. He confirmed that the results from the examinations showed she had deteriorated quite rapidly and dramatically. He prescribed a course of steroids. She had already had the tablet form which had not worked. She had to go into hospital during the day for intravenous steroid treatment, although she came home at night. This was a very depressing time for all of us as the symptoms were worsening and Stephanie had had no remission. Dr Dawson also confirmed that it was Multiple Sclerosis. While in the hospital Dr Dawson summoned me to speak to him in private. He told me that he was extremely worried about Stephanie and the way the she had deteriorated so rapidly. He was very concerned about the memory loss that Stephanie had been experiencing from the start. This made me extremely upset and worried. Why did this have to happen to someone who was so fit, healthy and loved life to the extreme? She had never smoked, taken drugs or had an excess of alcohol. She also ate extremely healthily. You could not fault her for that.

I started thinking back as to how this nightmare could have happened to someone so fit and healthy. She had suffered an ear infection that would not get better and had been prescribed two consecutive courses of antibiotics and then an antibiotic spray for the ear. She stopped training during this for about a week then went back to her training before she was fully recovered. She was due to compete in the National Championships in Scotland; we were advised by her coach that this was an extremely important event and even though Stephanie was not completely fit she should compete. In hindsight I realise now that I should have not let Stephanie swim. She travelled to Scotland by plane so that she would not be unduly tired for the championships. She did compete but her times were not good generally.

She was due to travel to China for the World School Games and needed a hepatitis and typhoid injection. I was not sure that she should have this injection due to her ear infection so I made an appointment to see Dr Jones. He assured me that as long as she didn't have a temperature she should go ahead and have the necessary injections, which she did. For me, this injection was the possible cause of Stephanie's MS. She never seemed to be well after that. She travelled to China and her times were still slower - she should have won but didn't.

One other factor in all this was stress. She was trying to do too much. She was training some mornings and every evening, attending school every day and having driving lessons. She was also trying to fit in seeing her boyfriend every day. She did not show any signs of stress but looking back on this time she must have been shattered. She should have possibly given up her A-levels and just concentrated on the swimming. It was a hard decision, which is why we just let her continue.

She was also having massive amounts of a sports drink which was provided by Bath University. In hindsight, once again, this contained high amount of phenalynanyne, which is not good for the nervous system.

I know that MS was not in her system before as she was so coordinated. She did ballet when she was five years old and was moved to an older class because she was so good. Her swimming strokes were always excellent - this could not have been achieved had she been un-coordinated. I know for sure that she has only recently been affected with this awful disease.

We heard about a new drug which made the symptoms of MS a third better and most patients who had used it had experienced a third fewer relapses. We asked about the possibility of this drug for Stephanie but, although she fitted the criteria perfectly, Wiltshire Health Authority did not prescribe the drug to its MS sufferers on the grounds of expense. Bath area did prescribe the drug to some of its sufferers. This was definitely a lottery.

I wrote to the Conservative MP for North Wiltshire, James Gray. He was very supportive and helpful, and sent me much detail concerning other sufferers in the county and the problems they had. He also sent me the latest details on the government's view on the drug. He invited Stephanie and us to lobby Parliament on 8 March 2000 with other MS sufferers. Stephanie had to decide on whether she wanted to go public with her MS. After much deliberation she decided that everyone who mattered to her knew of her condition and that by going public she may be helping to stop the unfairness of the postcode lottery. She told James Gray that she would join the campaign. During the following hours she was bombarded with journalists, radio station hosts etc. Although Stephanie was not at all prepared for the massive reaction she dealt with it very professionally. She was photographed and interviewed for the national papers as well as the locals. Her visit to Westminster was also televised. It amazed us all how well she dealt with all the questions as some were very distressing, and reminded her how well she did in the swimming world, even showing footage of her swimming days.

Stephanie made a very big impression for the MS cause. The *Bath Chronicle* newspaper decided they would back a campaign for Stephanie in order to stop the postcode lottery issue and hopefully influence the Wiltshire Health Authority to allow the drug that may help Stephanie's symptoms from deteriorating any further.

The campaign was extremely forceful and Stephanie's picture appeared daily in the *Chronicle*. The reporters always found news to accompany the pictures of postcode lottery issues. During this time Stephanie had many positive responses from people from all walks of life. Many of these responses lifted her spirits and made her feel that there were people out there who actually understood the way she felt. She had to wait many more months for the Wiltshire Health Authority to decide to prescribe the drug for Stephanie; months when the disease continued attacking her myelin sheath and months when Stephanie's condition was deteriorating at a rapid rate. If Stephanie had been prescribed the drug immediately who knows what differences it could have made - the drug may have been able to arrest the deterioration before it went too far.

After months of the *Bath Chronicle's* campaign we heard from Dr Dawson. He wanted to do all he could for Stephanie and was still very worried about her deterioration. He decided he would appeal to the Health Authority and to let them know that Stephanie's case should be treated as an exception due to the rapid deterioration and memory loss. We were pleased that he was backing Stephanie's case but I personally felt very frightened that he was still worried about Stephanie's condition.

I also wrote to the Health Authority's Appeal Panel before they met to let them know what kind of person Stephanie was before contracting this disease and some of the problems that she had encountered because of it. I told them how bright and active she was: always in the top eight in the year group, attending maths master classes for gifted mathematicians; winning Sports Personality of the Year; the national record holder in backstroke at 16 years old. I also told them how quick she was as a baby. How could a panel decide on Stephanie's future without knowing something about her?

The following few weeks were very difficult as we waited for the results of the panel. One morning, however, Dr Dawson phoned and wanted to speak to both Stephanie and I together. He told us that the Health Authority had decided to allow special exception in Stephanie's case because of her rapid deterioration. We were over the moon.

At last, Stephanie had been given a chance to move forward.

On hearing the results we had many and varied responses. Obviously the *Bath Chronicle* was overjoyed to hear the news. Some of Stephanie's fellow sufferers stopped talking to Stephanie and refused to come to a dinner that she had invited them to the following weekend. The television crews came around again to interview Stephanie and once again she was on local TV. She also appeared on the Trevor McDonald Show.

The MS nurse came around and demonstrated to us both how to give injections. Stephanie picked this up very quickly. I was not so good; I felt extremely unsure of giving my daughter injections. Stephanie had to give them to herself which she did this very well - I was very impressed.

She started on the Beteferon drug soon after that time. She was extremely well for the next couple of months, in fact she was almost back to normal.

Stephanie continued to do her A-levels at school and hardly had any absent days. She was continually worried that she was not retaining the information that was given. She went on, however, to take her A-levels - because she had problems reading the words (they would dart from one place to the next, and she had double vision) she was allowed a reader during the exams which I feel helped her confidence.

She then went on holiday to Tenerife with her sister and some friends. This was not a good time for Stephanie. She left behind part of her medication which we managed to send out on the next flight, but the immediate situation was extremely stressful for both Stephanie and Kristy. She also had her wallet stolen containing credit cards and cash. This was also a bad experience for her. All her symptoms reappeared with some new ones. Kristy was also very stressed trying to organise Stephanie during the holiday and they came back from there almost at each other's throats having been extremely good friends all their lives, Stephanie came back from holiday very tired and not very well at all.

During their holiday I collected both Stephanie's and Kristy's A-level exam results from school Stephanie had all but failed all of her A-levels but Kristy got a B in the module that Stephanie had failed on. This time was dreadful for Stephanie. She knew that she had revised all the work but she could not remember it when it was necessary. It was extremely frustrating for a girl who was so bright and intelligent to fail all her A-levels. I tried to reassure her that most people who had been through what Stephanie had would not have even sat them.

Shortly after returning from holiday we realised the new fridge was not working which meant that all Stephanie's medication had been spoiled. This was another worry for Stephanie although we later managed to recoup the money from the house insurance. It meant however that Stephanie had been injecting herself with useless medication. After this time Stephanie's symptoms worsened and she even mentioned using a wheelchair. I feel that it was because the medication was damaged. She also went on the pill as we established that her symptoms were very bad during her periods. The pill did seem to help but now there was another added development: Stephanie had put on weight especially around her stomach area.

She has continued to be depressed and frustrated. She decided that she would not take her anti-depressant medication any more, that she did not need it. Since this time Stephanie has been very bad tempered and unreasonable with the family. I spoke to my doctor who thought that she may have plaques on her emotions which could be affecting her moods.

While Stephanie was working for the local Co-op, she decided to accept a marketing job in Bristol. The first day she arrived home at 20:00 and the second she decided to quit due to the amount of walking the job involved. This had a very bad effect on Stephanie's moods - it must have felt as if she had another failure, although to me she had been brave to try something very new. The next few weeks were to be very difficult. She was desperate to find another job and spending even more time at home was not good for Stephanie. She felt her weight increased by the day. She was still on a low-fat diet so did not eat very much. She now cut even more food out of her diet in an attempt to reduce her weight but her weight continued to increase. She had more tests at the doctors to find out why this was so and she was referred to a nutritionist sometime in April. In the meantime she had to live with this. This latest failure of Stephanie's body seemed to affect Stephanie even more that the MS symptoms. I tried to stress to her the importance of eating to boost her body's defence system, but she was very worried that each spoonful would just increase the size of her stomach. The nutritionist confirmed that it was because her body was so used to a massive exercise regime and could not deal with this sudden inactivity. She said that her metabolism should correct itself in time.

Stephanie decided to embark on a computer course for the unemployed. She enjoyed doing this but some days would have problems getting to the bus stop as her legs would suddenly stop working. We tried to reassure her that we were just at the end of a phone. She felt, however, that her independence was gradually disappearing. During the course, a mature student on the course upset her by telling her that if she lost weight she would have a better chance of getting a job.

She decided to take driving lessons in an automatic. After several months she passed her test and we bought her a second hand automatic for her birthday. Some days she was not fit to drive due to her eyesight problems, but she at last felt that she had been successful at something.

Thank you, mum, for this document all about the nightmare from your eyes. You have always been there for me whenever the MS got in the way or even when my Sat Nav got lost!

You are amazing mum! Thank you for always being there for me! You took some of my pains and my worries away and there is no way I would have been able to do it on my own. Thank you for saving my life!

CHAPTER 37

Looking for an Answer

I wanted and needed to know what was making me sick. I had to find out why I was ill, what I had done wrong. I bought many large text books about neuroscience to try to learn why I had this illness. I thought these books were a fantastic buy even though they were very expensive. One of them was bound to tell me the reason I had MS and would tell me how to get over the disease. Once I had read all the chapters regarding the myelin sheath, stress and the reperfusion theory then I was sure I could find the cure for MS. I would then be able to continue my swimming career and be able to realise my dream of becoming the next Olympic gold medallist! Maybe all we need is someone with a fresh look on things who could see the cause and the cure of MS. I do know there are thousands of people trying to find the cure for MS and that they spend every day looking for and testing the information but I was certain I could find it just by looking through the text books! Every time I spotted a new text book about neuroscience or microbiology I bought it. The money I spent didn't seem as important as the reason for which I was buying the books. The money was irrelevant. The books were my answer, my cure and I needed all the help I could get. I needed to find my answers.

I spent a lot of time questioning a knowledgeable kinesiologist, Neil Harris, about the effects of stress on my brain and body. I was very interested in the reperfusion theory which basically discusses the idea of the body bringing oxygen and glucose to areas around the body after the supply has been stopped or slowed down in some way. I believe that this happens, that the body attacks itself as a normal response by your immune system, when you try to push yourself too hard and therefore overwork your body.

The blood supply of MS sufferers is known to carry less glucose and oxygen to their brain and spinal cord (the central nervous system) due to hypoperfusion, the decreased blood flow through an organ. This can cause neurodegeneration, the progressive loss of structure or function of neurons in the body's cells, and mitochondrial dysfunction. Mitochondria are organelles found in nearly every body cell and are the main power supply for the body, involved with producing Adenosine triphosphate (ATP) that is, basically, our energy. The dysfunction results in cell inactivity then ultimately cell death. As well as this ongoing process of neuro-degeneration, there are events which cause these glucose and oxygen levels to drop even lower such as an illness, stress, an infection etc. and when the event is over, the reperfusion cycle (the transfer of glucose and oxygen to specific areas around the body) begins again which is when we experience an 'MS attack'. So the incident occurs, you have the cold, infection or stress when the oxygen and glucose flow slows down and then the MS attack happens as a reaction to the lower oxygen and glucose supply. When the increased oxygen and glucose flow becomes available as you get better you experience the symptoms of the MS attack. This is why a lot of people say they had an infection or cold (or ear ache, in my case) before the MS symptoms started. I believe the hepatitis A injection I had was my MS trigger.

I had never been to the doctors before I got sick with the MS: why had it suddenly changed? I demanded information about the injection that I had before I went to China. I searched in my text books and on the internet to get all the information I could about hepatitis A, formaldehyde, which was the stabiliser used in my injection, and aluminium hydroxide which was the makeup of the injection. I found out about formaldehyde in particular as I thought this could be the possible link to MS. Formaldehyde is made up of double bonds to a single hydrogen atom, and single oxygen atoms, which are normally O_2, two oxygen atoms bonded together. There must be something not quite right here. H_2O Hydrogen and oxygen bonded together makes water but then H_2O_2 (adding one more oxygen) you get bleach. How violent is that extra or that single oxygen atom? Oxygen is therefore a key factor! What would turn my body against itself? Could it be too much oxygen?

When I am training I have to make sure that my body remembers to breathe. I will turn my head in anticipation of the breath but then seem to forget the breathing part. It is pretty annoying because then I have to breathe again straight away which slightly ruins my routine! I therefore have to consciously remember to breathe!

I was currently swimming a two hour session early in the mornings as well as working a forty hour week in a wonderful credit control post, but I still decided that I had to do evening accountancy courses as well, to cover myself in things to do so that I don't have to worry about the future or to realise the pain in my arms and legs. All I needed to do was to pass my exams as quickly as possible and then, even if I lose my memory eventually, I would have all the qualifications. It's a bit like swimming, really. I used to be the British record holder so even if I can't swim anymore I still have that! I am sure that when I am older and more disabled all I will have to think about is that British record, about being an accountant and about being the best I could have been. The fact that by then I could have lost it all is pretty irrelevant because I would be living in the care of my mother or possibly someone I love if I ever find that someone. I would still be trying to do everything I can. Being happy has always been important in my life so even if I get very sick or lose my ability to see or speak, I have to stay happy. MS thrives off depression and every time I am unhappy the MS shows its ugly face but if I can continue doing things I like doing and trying not to worry about the future I am certain I can lock the MS behind those bars I had envisaged all those years ago when I wrote the poem 'MS - My War' (see chapter 31). Finally I believe I can keep the MS away, I can be strong, I can be the winner.

Me against the MS, and I am in charge. Stephanie vs MS. One nil!

CHAPTER 38

Dear Ronan Keating

Stephanie Millward
Box,
Nr. Corsham,

Dear Ronan Keating,

I have written this note to say a million 'Thank yous' to you, Westlife and Boyzone. (Could you pass on the note for me please?)

You have all helped me come to terms with an incurable, debilitating disease that I have been diagnosed with. I am currently 19 years old but when I was 18 and 4 days I was told that I had MS. This ruined my life but your songs have given me hope and the strength to carry on with life. Your songs have **always** given me hope.

Before I got the illness, I was an international swimmer. I used all the songs as ways of winning. I used to listen to the songs before I raced and, consequently, I almost always won! I had to give up training for the Olympics when I got MS. This came as a shock as I had always swam for at least 20 hours a week. I was left with nothing to fill my time. I listened to all your CDs a million times.

Through listening to the songs I found that every song

related to my life in some way. When I listen to sad songs I think of my life as a swimmer before the MS. Your words make me smile because I think of what my life was like and I feel very proud of myself and everything that I have already achieved! The words now give me the strength to fight my illness. They help me look forward to my life even with the disease.

I wrote a poem when I was feeling very ill and upset with life which was printed in the local newspaper. Many people said that they had been moved by my words and someone asked if they could make it into a song.

The song will be released as a chart single within the next few months. I am not looking for any success with it; I just hope that some money can be raised for the MS Society. The song is called 'Paying the Price'.

Thank you so much for helping me to rebuild my crushed life. You are my lifesavers and I wish you all the luck in the world.

Thank you.

Yours sincerely,
Stephanie Millward

so why can't everything else die now too? My dad leaving was just proof that everything had gone wrong. Proof, that the MS was not just an incorrect diagnosis and proof that I was indeed going to get sicker and sicker, end up blind and in a wheelchair. Bad things come in threes apparently. The MS, the end of my swimming life and the divorce. It was already written, it was always going to happen.

Whose fault was it? For years I blamed myself because I had got sick but I realise now it was actually nobody's fault; it is just the way life goes sometimes. Many people reading this chapter will know how hard things get with divorce or family break-ups. It wrecks your life. Someone always has to be blamed so I took it upon myself to be that person and everyone seemed happy with this outcome. They separated because I got sick. I told many people that it was my fault and they all listened with sympathetic ears. I know now that it was not my fault and that it was always going to happen eventually. It wasn't right for my mum and dad, I was just the catalyst.

My home life had been bliss as everything had been perfect, or that is what I had thought, but in reality things were obviously not good and hadn't been for a while. My illness was just the start, I thought, for the end of my relationship with my dad. It took me a while to realise but it wasn't the end of our relationship, it was just the start my dad and I having to look at each other in a different. It was often hard to start conversations when he was so far away from me but time seemed to heal the space between us. Over the time and the years I have learned to deal with these strange, unnatural obstacles that have come before me and those that have got in the way of my dad and me. His new partner was especially hard to take. He had chosen his path and I had to find mine yet. I needed so much help from him; his words were just not enough. He probably knew that too. I needed him at that point in time but he couldn't come back to help. We have muddled on for years with sparse conversations and infrequent get-togethers, some of which have been very strained, as you can imagine. The slightest disagreement or disapproval of my actions causes great pain to the both of us. I try, he tries; we both try. There is now another person in his life. I still feel that I should be the only person but I am not five anymore and he is not the young dad protecting me or saving me when I fell into the pool. While it was easy to blame his new partner, it was not her fault.

Our relationship is much better now even though he has moved about five hundred miles away from me. We have come to a silent agreement that as long as we are both happy then we can live our lives in peace and we can be happy for each other. I believe now that my dad's partner is keeping him happy and he knows that swimming is back in my life and I am now doing exactly what I should have been doing approximately ten years ago when I first got sick. We are living our lives in an almost calm serenity and it must be the best way possible. Hopefully my dad will be as happy as I want him to be and will grow old content. The bright yellow summer flowers at the end of a dreadfully dark, cold winter.

Good luck, Dad! I will love you forever, wherever you may be.

CHAPTER 40

My Past

Please don't let me forget it,
I had such a perfect life
It was so amazing
Myself so outstanding
Keep memories of the past.

A life to be proud of
I need to remember my past
A need for the old me
Scared of the new me
I was worthy of a royal
A life always to be proud of.

Why is it over?
Why did it stop?
I need all the strength,
The determination, the hope,
Needing to rebuild my dreams,
To fix all my shattered hopes.

CHAPTER 41

Spring, 23rd January 2003

My best friend, maybe my only friend. Spring had been there for me whenever I needed her and she didn't want anything but my love in return.

I was in my bedroom watching the television when Spring, my Yorkshire terrier, came up to me, kissing me and being very loving. I told her how much I loved her and thanked her for being so wonderful to and for me. Spring was perfect and I hope I made her feel good.

Spring left the room and about ten minutes later I heard Kristy scream. I knew what had happened even before I saw her motionless body on the kitchen floor. Nicholas came running in and on seeing Spring on the floor he turned away. Kristy and I cried; we cried for a part of our family, for an amazing friend, cried for the grieving pain in our hearts. Spring had been there for me every day since the start of my MS and before that when we first got her she was my playmate, jumping pony jumps that I had set up in the garden. She was so incredible for us; she was sweet-tempered, good, perfect. After seeing me that day, Spring had gone to each other member of the family (apart from Paul, who was in Australia) just to say goodbye and I love you before she went to her favourite place, the kitchen, where she lay down and died. Even though she is no longer here I often feel that she is still by my side. The strength she has given to me over the past four years with the MS and the eight years before that will stay with me for the rest of my life.

Spring spent a lot of her time barking at the fish in the pond and often jumped in the pond to catch the fish before leaving them on the side of the pond in the grass waiting for someone to push it back in. Spring seemed to love the pond and the river at the bottom of the garden and so this is where we scattered her ashes, leaving her exactly where she would have liked to have been left. The memories will remain around the pond and the river forever even though we have moved house now. These memories are printed in my mind and whenever I am feeling ill or unhappy I just need to remember my past when Spring and I would run around the garden jumping all the jumps and then sitting down on the sofa afterwards together, exhausted but happy. While a child I never needed to suck my thumb and I only used a dummy when I was bad tempered but now I get comfort from my family and from my pets; each of them had the ability to take my mind off any bad thing that is happening to me at that point in my life. Spring was wonderful for me and she helped me to come to terms with the fact that I have an illness, probably for the rest of my life, and the only thing I can do is to enjoy my life to the best I can.

I hope everybody has someone like Spring in their life. She will be forever a strength even though she is no longer here with me. In my mind I feel as though she is always there when I need her, always there to guide me, always smiling and always happy.

CHAPTER 42

Learning to Stand,
21st October 2005

Dear Diary

I went to the gym today to try to lose some weight and all she said to me was that I needed to be re-inducted on the machines because it had been six years since I had last been and they had had new machines. Don't people know how much I am hurting psychologically as well as physically? Why did she have to be so cruel? If I had reached the Olympics she wouldn't have been so mean to me. Why does she have to kick me when she knows how badly I have already fallen?

I went home and cried. It makes the whole thought of trying to lose weight that much harder. They must know that I used to work on those machines all the time and that I was very good and very strong at one point, but six years? Have six years gone by that quickly? What have I done with my life? Nothing. Oh, six years is an incredibly long time. I decided against going to the gym but instead my mum found me a personal trainer called John, who on paper looked perfect for me. Hopefully he could help me. I was eating just about nothing and piling the weight on so I was obviously doing something wrong. My doctors said that my body was just confused because it had been working so hard and now my body was able to do just about nothing. My poor body didn't know what it had done wrong. Me neither, I thought. Me neither.

John was a nice man. When he first saw me struggle to walk he didn't look down on me or speak to me as if I was very young or not very clever. He stayed positive and happy and said that he would help me get back on my feet. He was a kind person and I enjoyed trying to stand and trying to sit on a ball which I found very difficult, and then when John asked me to lift one of my feet off the ground the obvious happened and I found myself lying flat on the mat! John cost me £25 per half-hour but this was money well spent as in the end I was able to sit on the ball and raise my feet. Then I was able to walk putting me heel down first - heel toe, heel toe!

I had my sessions with John in Victoria Park in Bath which is a stunning location and when John asked me what my end goal was I said that it had been an Olympic gold medal originally but now it was being able to run again. After work we walked, jogged, then ran together. With me losing weight and getting stronger I was beginning to feel that I was back in control. I was enjoying my life again, I was almost well: I felt I could do anything. I was over the moon that I could run again even if it was holding onto somebody else's arm. My eyesight was not wonderful and movement proved difficult (well, actually close to impossible) when I was going faster than a walk.

I looked into running/walking the Bath half-marathon. Maybe I could run this and get loads of sponsorship money for MS. This was an unreal expectation but Sonia Bush my good friend told me about a friend of hers, Caroline, who was also hoping to run the half-marathon. I met her and we went for a few runs but unfortunately on one of the runs I fell flat on my face cutting my hands and knees and I realised that running was probably a little too difficult for me at that moment. I could run approximately four hundred metres so the thirteen mile run would have been quite a long way for me! Oh well! Me and my unreal expectations, but at least I lost a little bit of weight and made some friends in the process.

I tried to go for a walk every day, pushing the distance covered each and every time. It started with learning to stand and balance myself, then learning to move each foot. Heel, toe, heel, toe. I kept putting the toe down first because of my balance issues which obviously kept showing their faces. Just one more step, Stephanie. One more step. I found it exciting that I kept going that little bit further. I was getting stronger! Five metres turned into twenty metres which turned into one hundred metres! I felt stronger with every step!

It is funny what life offers us sometimes. I was walking around Jolly's one day and I saw a man trying to sell massaging chairs. I thought, well he can try to sell me the chair if he wants and I will just rest my legs in the chair for a while, so I did! The man, Jonathan Payne, came over and did his sales stuff and then we got chatting. He asked me what I did and I asked him what he did other than sell chairs. Jonathan was a singer/songwriter which interested me as I had written the poem/song Paying the Price. In the end we went to the coffee shop and he bought me a cup of tea and a scone with strawberry jam! We became friends and he said he would love to write a song about my life and my journey so far. We met on numerous occasions working together to put this song together. The song is called 'Everyone all around me' and it is a song about learning to do all the easy things first: standing, walking, talking, and then eventually finding love at the end of the fight. It is a story about my life in simple terms and I enjoyed writing it with Jonathan.

'And with everyone all around me I'm not standing on my own, I know I can make it, know I can take it, know I can find my way back home.'

While writing this song and trying to get fit I decided to start a course in Tai Kwon Do at the local sports centre (the Springfield centre). It was two one-hour sessions a week which I loved. I gained a lot of core strength and it helped in every way possible. I also decided to go and ask the coach at Chippenham ASC if I could help teach the children who swam there. In the end I was teaching many youngsters to swim and I loved offering them something I used to be so good at.

I was taking one of my accountancy courses at Chippenham College and teaching at Chippenham ASC when I decided to start swimming on Sunday morning with my wonderful friend, Sonia Bush. We had a great time at Bath University pool and, although it was where I swam when I was able, I enjoyed swimming with Sonia. We both got stronger appreciating the swimming and enjoying losing weight with both of us wondering why swimming didn't help with the size of one's stomach! Oh well, sit-ups are not too difficult I suppose. Sonia also taught swimming as a job and she took me to teach the children with her which I really enjoyed!

While I was swimming one Sunday I saw the Melksham ASC team come over and get ready for their swims. I went and introduced myself, telling Dave Pegg, the coach at Melksham ASC, that I used to swim for Corsham ASC but got sick. Dave knew who I was and he knew about my illness and as he was a school teacher he knew which words to say to me that wouldn't make me cry with the recognition of what had happened! Dave introduced me to another John who was also a swimming coach for Melksham. John listened to my story and watched me swim, commenting on how neat my strokes were even without the training. He mentioned then that I should either get back into swimming or come and teach at Melksham. I did the latter and started coaching at both Chippenham and Melksham, and working, and taking my accountancy course, and doing Tai Kwon Do - life was pretty busy and stopped me thinking about the MS! The Tai Kwon Do was brilliant because it taught me how to balance and how to concentrate on my core body strength. The teaching was wonderful because it reminded me how much I loved swimming and how much I had learned as a swimmer. I loved trying to teach the children to be as good as I had been!

The Multiple Sclerosis society was a point of interest for me because it was a way I could find out what the best and worst outcomes for me were. Does anyone else get through MS without needing a wheelchair? I used mine only very occasionally, hoping each time that I would never sit in it again! I always walked by the walls ready to put my arm out for support when I stumbled or wobbled.

One morning I received a letter from the MS Society inviting me to go to Copenhagen to give a speech about my life in front of a number of medical students. I was very excited as they were going to pay for all my expenses, and my mum and her then-partner, Mervyn Potter, were allowed to come with me. The flight was fantastic and I loved everything about this event. Copenhagen was an exciting place and I met so many people which was very good experience for me. I had to do two speeches: one as a practice, and the second as the real thing in front of a large number of people. The practice came and I had a few photos to show everyone. I had to touch the screen and the picture would come up. My mum and her partner were sitting in front of me but towards the back of the small group that were in to watch the practice. I started my speech:

'Am I SM, Stephanie Millward, or am I MS, the girl with Multiple Sclerosis?' The S and the M letters turned around perfectly!

I kept on going with the story watching the tears falling from the eyes of everyone in front of me and I stayed strong. 'Do not give up yet. They are only words, they have already happened, they will not hurt you now.'

'Unfortunately my life didn't go the way I had planned but I am staying strong hoping that the cure will be found.' It was only at this point that I saw the tears falling fast and strong from my mum's eyes.

'Um.' My mum's tears hit me hard in my heart. 'Remember the good things that have happened and trust that the bad things are all in the past.'

Everybody clapped and I felt exhausted with too many emotions and too many feelings. My mum was crying in front of me.

After the practice I was a little apprehensive about the real thing. Everyone had said how well it had gone but it had hurt me emotionally - I felt exhausted. The real speech came and a nice man said he would click the pictures for me, which was great except he didn't do it quite as well as planned and was late with the majority of the screens! The speech was good and this time my mum was ready for my words and so didn't cry which made it easier for me as I didn't feel her pain too. The trip to Copenhagen was a wonderful experience!

Everyone all around me

Sung by Jonathan Payne with words by Stephanie Millward and Jonathan Payne

Learning to stand, learning to be who I am,
Learning to walk, learning to walk where I want
And with everyone all around me, I'm not standing on my own
And with everyone all around me, I know I can make it, know I can take it know I can find my way back home.
Learning to stand, learning to be who I am.

Learning to run, learning to run to who I've become,
Learning to breathe, breathing the wind that sets me free.
And with everyone all around me, I can run a million miles.
And with everyone all around me, I know I'm beginning and I know I'm winning, nobody knows how hard I've tried.
Learning to run, learning to become.

When I cross that finish line there's a medal that is mine and it's gold every time,
If I learn to love, so I'm learning to love.
And with everyone all around me, I can run a million miles,
And with everyone all around me, I know I'm beginning but I know I'm winning nobody knows how hard I've tried.
Learning to run, learning to become.
Learning to stand, learning to be who I am!

This song that John and I wrote together now be found on myspace which is very exciting.
https://myspace.com/jonathanpaynesongs/music/song/everyone-all-around-me27283535-27084720

The words are an exclamation of all the feelings I was having at that point in time but now I have re-learned to stand, re-learned to walk and have found my way back home or at least to a place in this world that makes me happy and strong. Step by step I got stronger. Every step is another mile in my heart, every step is a million hurdles I have had to fight and have yet to fight. Everyone is offered something in their own lives, often obstacles that are near impossible to get over. Everyone has the option of either grasping the obstacle with open arms and a huge smile on their face seeing it as an opportunity or they can fight it and see all the negatives. Thankfully, I chose to stand and fight and I can see the importance of each and every step.

Learning or rather re-learning to stand and move was so important for me. Every step counts, every step matters, believe it and enjoy it!

CHAPTER 43

Holistic Medicine

There is another type of medical treatment that can be used for MS sufferers, or any form of illness, other than the conventional medical treatments. This is holistic medicine and may include the following: acupuncture; osteopathy; homeopathy; aromatherapy; applied kinesiology; reflexology; hypnotherapy; massage. Holistic medicine followed the belief that the whole body includes the mind, the body and the spirit.

Normally, the body is in perfect balance but whenever somebody is ill, it means that there is an imbalance in that person's life which may be just a worry or a stress. Healers often believe that there are no 'incurable' diseases and that any condition can be improved by bringing the body back into the correct balance and getting rid of any possible blockages in the body's usual flow. It is also believed that the body is able to heal itself if all the external conditions are correct. Holistic healers can make your life better if you can believe that they can improve your life. It all rests with the power of your mind and your ability to trust your healers!

My personal healing

I have found that holistic healing is a brilliant form of treatment for my MS. It has offered me hope, raised the positive awareness that there are other ways of helping myself to recover from an illness and has helped me to come to terms with my life and what it has offered me at this moment in time.

It all sounds a little bit unreal but I have found the holistic healing in the form of Reiki to be very helpful. Reiki is a word used to describe a system of natural healing. It is a Japanese technique for stress reduction and relaxation that also promotes healing. It is administered by 'laying on hands' and is based on the idea that an unseen life-force energy flows through us and is what causes us to be alive. If one's life-force energy is low then one is more likely to get sick or feel stress, and if it is high, we are more capable of being happy and healthy.

I think that it could help anyone. It is extraordinary! My brilliant healers were Peter and Linda Woodgate and my incredible naturopath healer is Neil Harris and his wonderful partner, Ibby Wallace. Each healer in their own special way has been standing by my side while I have struggled with this illness and each one has offered me advice and comfort. They have also offered me hope and have given me the ability to help myself whenever I am in pain. When a person has a headache they cup their hands over their head and the warmth from your hands 'heals' the pain in your head. I do the same when I have pins and needles and whenever I have pain in my limbs and it works every time. Our bodies are incredible! I remained good friends with Neil and Ibby when Linda and Peter Woodgate moved to New Zealand. They helped me remain positive and kept me smiling whenever something went wrong. Ibby wrote loads of amazing manuscripts which should be turned into books for people to enjoy. One of the fantastic presents Ibby gave to me was a poem written by her all about me. Her poem is called Mermaid and it is incredible. Please find Mermaid in chapter 44. Unfortunately, cancer attacked and won the battle with Ibby but I still believe she is watching me smiling. Angels are everywhere!

Two useful things I use to help to rid myself of the pain I experience with MS are written below. If you suffer from pain give them a go to see if the pain is eased or just goes away!

Firstly, I basically rely on the power of the mind. Pain is all in the mind so it is your mind telling you there is pain somewhere where really there is nothing. You have to concentrate on clearing the paths in your body. Send or imagine sending white light all the way through your body, through all your veins and this light will clear all the paths and stop all the pain. Let the light run out of the bottom of your feet and with it all your pain.

Fatigue is much the same. Chronic Fatigue or general tiredness can be all the MS or other illness you have. Watch and record how much exercise or movement you do in a day. Should you be tired? If so, rest, but if not make yourself move and tell your brain that you are not tired. Convince yourself you feel no pain and no tiredness.

Secondly, is by squeezing your fists. Whenever it all gets too much for you squeeze both your fists and think you are resetting your programme. Breathe in, squeeze your fists as hard as you can then breathe out, and release the tension. All your stresses will go out through your hands while you are breathing out! You will then be ready to address the world again!

Another form of therapy I find very useful is hypnotherapy. Hypnotherapy is a form of psychotherapy used to create unconscious change in the patient in the form of new responses, thoughts, attitudes, behaviours or feelings. It is undertaken with a subject in hypnosis. My hypnotherapist, Andy Milton, is a good friend of mine and we chat for hours about ways to change the world for the better. Andy says that he watches for a number of things when he is hypnotising somebody as a person who is hypnotised displays certain unusual characteristics and propensities compared with a non-hypnotised subject, most notably heightened suggestibility and responsiveness. Andy often noted the flickering eyes when I was walking down the steps in my mind to the hypnotised area in my brain. It was an incredible feeling and such a useful life-changing possibility that would allow anyone the ability to progress from a standstill position to enormous levels of success! Thank you Andy for everything you helped me with! Andy and I did a lot of work on my underwater kick when leaving the blocks and off the wall at a turn. We imagined the race and we went through the motions in my mind making an extra point of strong kicks off the wall and extra power similar to a dolphin moving off the walls! The image of a dolphin or that of a mermaid swimming within me helps to promote me to swim faster! The power of the mind is incredible!

CHAPTER 44
Mermaid

Chapter the First

I

Myth of the ocean,
Nymph of the sea.
Half fish, half sprite,
Aquatic faerie.
Perfectly formed
From skin to scale,
Strangely conjoined
From flesh to tail.
Cutting through water,
Streamlined and sleek,
With powerful thrust
And perfect physique.
A swish
Through a swirl,
Diving deep
For a pearl.
From surface to seabed
In descending spin,
Countering currents
By the flick of a fin.

II

Sea goddess
From head to hip,
Extraordinary fish
From navel to tip.
All human above
With voluptuous torso
Merged in iridescence
To the tail below.
All mother-of-pearl
And aquamarine.
A coil and flip
Too fleet to be seen.
Rarely glimpsed
By human sight,
The mermaid swims
Too fast for light.
Preserving her myth,
Her legend intact.
Is she fiction?
Or is she fact?

III

True apparition
Or fanciful lie?
A corner sighting
From a sailor's eye
Of a beautiful,
Fishtailed female form,
Diving through the surge
Of an oncoming storm.
A water angel
Who will save his life

By guiding the clipper
Through the broil and strife
Of angry squall
And hurricane wind
Until the tempest abates
And the waves rescind.
Are those two blue eyes
And long golden hair
Merely the figment
Of a sailor's prayer?

Chapter the Second

I

I know a mermaid
Alive on dry land,
With two shapely legs
On which she can stand.
But her golden hair
And sea blue eyes
Betray her
Lower limbed disguise
As she walks her way
Upright and able,
Through her own
Human fable.
A parallel story
Of life and line
Already well known
Beneath the brine
Where the water kingdom's
Legend of old
Is a favourite yarn
Frequently told.

II

A tale that
I must now relate
To put an end
To all debate.
A narrative bound
To astonish all
Delivered to excite,
Intrigue and enthral
As cynicism melts
Into sheer delight
Where sceptic and romantic
Inadvertently unite
Under the orators
Word-woven spell.
The magic that logic
Fails to quell,
Rendering an audience
Unable to resist
The undeniable truth
That mermaids exist.

III

Once upon a mermaid
In a kingdom marine,
Far from terra firma
In the deep blue and green,
Where choral gardens
And seaweed sway
Set a scenic backdrop
For a theatrical display
Of a shoal's precise
And unanimous concern

As stripe and colour
Twitch and turn
Beneath patrolling shadows
Of long-tailed doom
As rhomboid harbinger
Stingrays loom
And omen to misfortune
Is but a fin's breadth delay
As danger's ever presence
Paves Calamity's way.

Chapter the Third

I

Unaware of Calamity's
Impending whims,
Our underwater heroine
Gaily swims
Up and down,
Along and across,
Happily ignorant
Of future loss.
The world is her oyster,
That oyster is supreme,
Its pearl of circumference
And radiance extreme.
Her prospects tremendous,
Her reputation grown
As the fastest mermaid
Ever known.
Able to swim
At a pace so bold,
Passing bronze and silver
To certain gold.

II

But on her way
To The Great Mermaid Race
Calamity struck
And stole her place.
Before the contest
Had even begun,
Misfortune competed
And consequently won
By injecting poison
From a sea urchin's spine
Into her tail
So sleek and fine.
Her perfect speed
Stopped dead in its tracks.
Her mirror to the future
Criss-crossed by cracks,
Poised to shatter
What should have been
And reflect that loss
In each smithereen.

III

Each shard embedded
In a broken dream
Unravelling to the silence
Of her internal scream
As pain explodes
Beyond threshold's scope
And the poison spreads
Dissolving all hope
To leave in its wake
An unforeseen dread

As her arms and tail
Turn to lead,
Anchoring our champion
To depths unknown
Where her heart aches
In its breaking zone
But somehow resists
That final tear
Of hopelessness
And utter despair.

Chapter the Fourth

I

A courageous heart beats
At a pace so bold
Passing bronze and silver
To certain gold.
Our mermaid possesses
Such a heart
Forestalling despondency
With a clear head start,
Outpacing the sea urchin's
Toxic traces,
Putting disappointments
Back in their places,
She flicks her tail
And starts to swim
Out from under
Calamity's whim.
A golden resolve
Misfortune forgot
From molten flow
To pure ingot.

II

Our heroine radiates
A love and joy
The injected contagion
Can never destroy.
She laughs, she frolics,
She jumps, she dives.
Her smile lights up
A thousand lives
As shoals about turn
In her direction
And dolphins provide
Their playful protection
To an untainted spirit
The venom cannot quell
As she rides the seahorse
Or the turtle's shell
And all acknowledge
Her magical presence,
All mother-of-pearl
And iridescence.

III

While her golden heart
Is worn within,
The once begun
Must again begin,
To capture the gold
She will wear without,
To continue the quest
And quash any doubt
That she is a mermaid
Of some renown,

Destined to wear
The laurel crown
And a gold medallion
Around her neck,
A prize the sea urchin
Can no longer wreck
As smote but undaunted
She reclaims her place
And swims towards
The Great Mermaid Race.

Isabel Mary Wallace Copyright 2009
For Stephanie Millward

CHAPTER 45

Kristy

Kristy Suzanne Millward, my special, perfect sister. She is like the star on the top of any Christmas tree. She is wonderful and brilliant and almost everybody loves her.

At this point in my life I just felt jealous, absolutely and completely jealous of her. She was getting everything and I was getting absolutely nothing. She had a special boyfriend called Sam Wade as well as loads of other friends. I didn't even have one mate. Her friends kept her busy, inviting her out on holidays and days out. I stayed in my room with Spring crying. Kristy has always been my best friend and we got on so well but when my MS arrived everything changed. My life went drastically downhill and Kristy's kept going up. My tears, my sadness came but she never stopped laughing. Every time I came out of my room I looked for Kristy and she was often with Sam, in her room. At least I suppose she was close by. Could they see my hurt? Could they see my pain? They didn't seem to. I often carried a book under my arm about Multiple Sclerosis searching, maybe even looking for a comment. The comment never came. I often went into Kristy's room just to talk to someone. I couldn't really have a good conversation with Spring as I never got a reply. I was jealous of everything Kristy had and did and the immense pain in my heart deepened. Every time I saw her she was happy with her life; my life was desperately sad and lonely and sitting in my room was very miserable. Alone with Spring. Kristy tried to include me in almost all that she did but things didn't always work out because inevitably my inability to walk compromised her every effort to include me. Kristy went on with her life as best she could. Her AS-levels and then her A-levels were her priority and my illness was something she had yet to accommodate for and to fully understand. Kristy was very hard-working and studied for her exams very intensely, making sure she would get the results she wanted.

The connection between Kristy and Sam as a couple coincided with the start of my MS, they met and I got sick at the same time. This seemed to be at the complete opposite ends of the scale of happiness. On one end there was my sister with the devoted love of Sam and on the other end I was being brutally abused by the disease Multiple Sclerosis. My sister had no idea of the pain I was going through with her relationship going so well. I found it hard to deal with but was pleased that Kristy had found someone so wonderful, someone that made her smile. I wanted someone to help me smile. Someone just to hug me occasionally, someone to say hi, someone, anyone.

Kristy was so perfect with a stunning face, good at everything, had loads of friends and had Sam: her life was amazing. Kristy has always been special and extraordinary and she had everything. I wanted a Sam. Someone strong and devoted and who loved me immensely as Sam did Kristy. Kristy and Sam took on the roles of Barbie and Ken for me with perfect life that I could only dream about. The toy dolls that could do the things you dreamed of doing. Give me a chance. I wanted to be Barbie just for a while. Maybe one day Ken will find me and I will be happy again. I will be strong and comfortable. I will be best friends with Kristy again like we used to be, maybe. Yes, I want to be Barbie for a while. I want to be happy again. I want Kristy to be happy too as she is incredible and amazing and I am so proud of her, but can I have a tiny bit of good luck too as this dark life of mine is so hard to bear? Just a minute being Barbie, just a moment of happiness.

CHAPTER 46

Adrian McHugh – My Angel, 3rd March 2005

Dear Diary

'I am your Sam!' Adrian had said. 'I am your Sam.'

'Can you read my mind? Those were the words I had been looking for. Adrian must have known that this is exactly what I wanted. Sam had been so strong and so perfect for Kristy; I had wanted a Sam. Can he read my mind? Is he perfect for me? Is he an angel?

Looking into his eyes I questioned how much he knew about what I was thinking. How did he know I wanted a Sam for myself? How did he know I was looking for a special friend to help me live my life the way I wanted to? How did he read my mind just at that moment? Does he know how much I am hurting? Does he want to fix my broken heart? Is he going to use me or leave me? Is he my angel?

Adrian seemed to be everything I needed and whether we were in the gym struggling to run for a whole ten minutes or whether it was me trying to teach Adrian to breathe properly when he was swimming, we enjoyed each other's company so much. Has God sent me Adrian to try to help me out? Is Adrian the reply to all those prayers I have said or the answer to all the questions I have asked? Adrian must be an angel; nobody else is this nice.

I wanted everyone to like me even though I had MS so I acted as the person they wanted me to be. I tried very hard to try to be happy but there were so many bad things happening to me and so many bad people I had thought were my friends. I was used by selfish people who took rather than gave but when I met Adrian he just gave and gave. Adrian convinced me that people liked me because they liked me and I didn't have to do anything to earn that.

I was very angry that my life had been stolen from me and I was left like a broken wreck. I really wanted someone to share my pain and Adrian watched and learned from every time I broke down. He knew what to do and what to say to put a smile back on my face. He saw the broken heart, he felt the wounded tears, he wanted to lift me up where I had fallen, to give me the strength to help rebuild my life and to make my poems happy and uplifting rather than depressed and hurtful. He wanted to dry my tears and to kiss all my pain away. Adrian could see a kind, warm and gentle girl under all the tears and pain and every time I burst out crying it gave Adrian a chance to try to help me. I needed a friend but instead, like all the fairy stories and like our dreams, I found true love.

I was very apprehensive to tell Adrian I had MS. I expected him to stay away after I had told him, like everyone else had, but instead he stayed and we grew stronger and stronger.

I had met Adrian originally in the most perfect place. In a swimming pool! A friend of mine, Mike Cox, with whom I swam in the early morning sessions, asked me to teach his friend Adrian how to swim so he can do a triathlon. I obviously agreed and went over to say hi and introduce myself! In the end, Adrian helped me in the gym and I taught him to swim. When he didn't go away after I had told him I had MS I grew more confident that MS was not such a bad thing. I am a nice person and people were putting the MS first. The MS should always be put behind. It is not controlling my life anymore. I had been trapped by the MS and Adrian has made me realise that anything is still achievable and that I am in charge as opposed to the illness being in control.

I had lent money to a few male friends and they had walked away

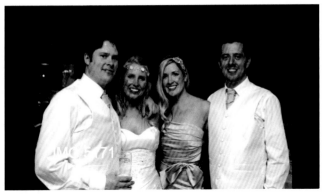

Paul, Stephanie, Kristy and Nicholas Millward at Stephanie's wedding.

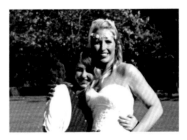

Stephanie with Amy Jelinek Stephanie's amazing friend and star supporter!

Stephanie, Tigs, Heather and Ken Marshall.

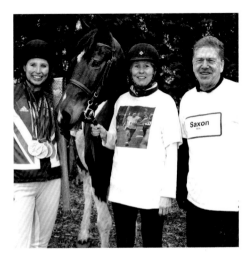

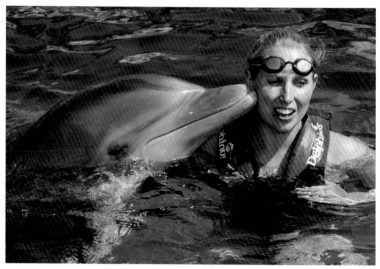

Stephanie being kissed by a dolphin.

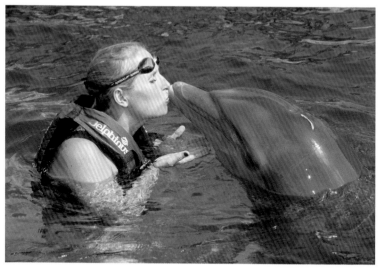

Stephanie kissing the dolphin back!

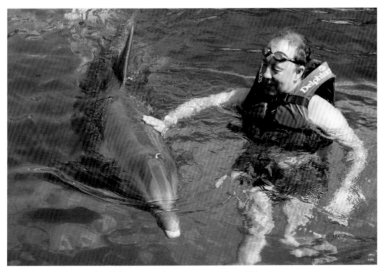

Adrian stroking the dolphin. (He was scared stiff!)

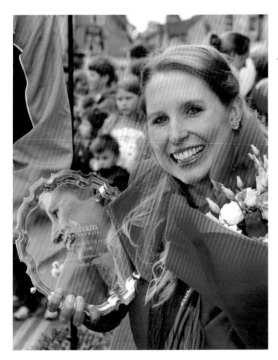

Stephanie with her silver salver and flowers on receiving the Freedom of Corsham honour.

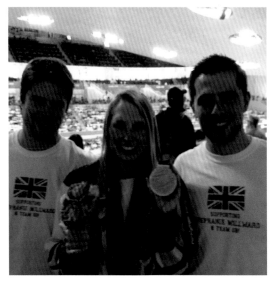

Paul, Stephanie and Nicholas Millward at London Paralympics Games after winning the silver medal for 100m backstroke.

Adrian and Stephanie at Buckingham Palace for the Queens garden party.

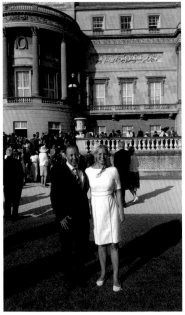

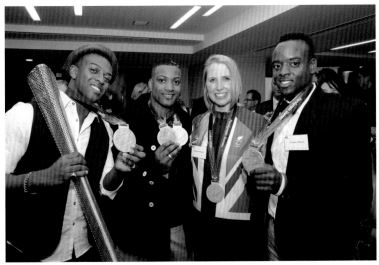

JLS (or some of it) wearing Stephanie's medals! (Amazing guys!)

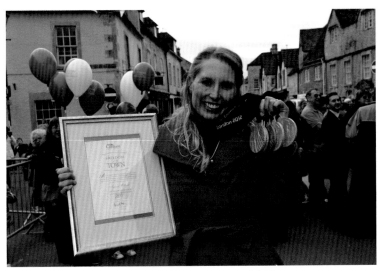

Stephanie receiving Freedom of Corsham honour 2013.

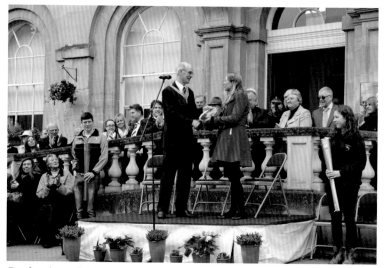

Stephanie receiving Freedom of Corsham honour 2013.

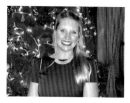

Stephanie and Nicholas Millward in Jeddah after Stephanie's three little pigs ballet dance.

Stephanie at BBC Sports Personality of the Year Awards.

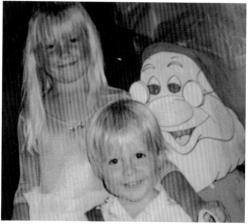

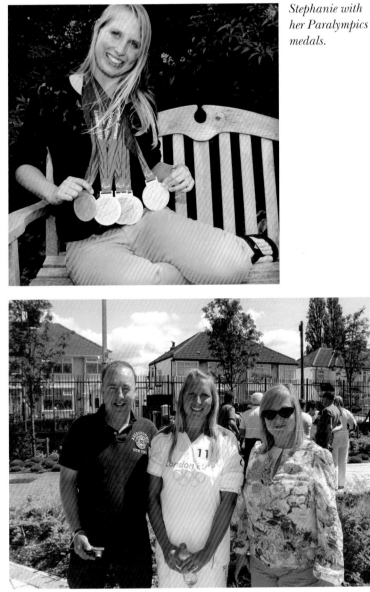

Stephanie with her Paralympics medals.

Adrian McHugh, Stephanie and Linda Millward getting ready to carry the Olympic Torch.

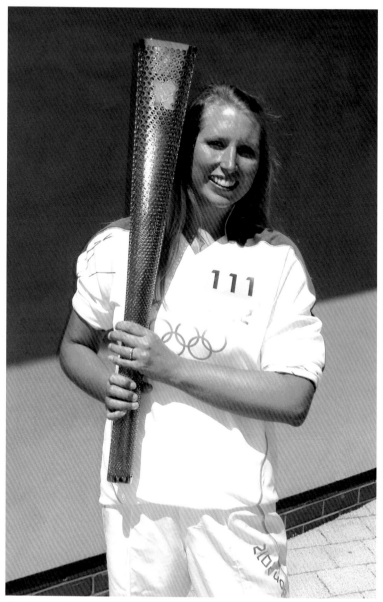

Stephanie after carrying the Olympic Torch.

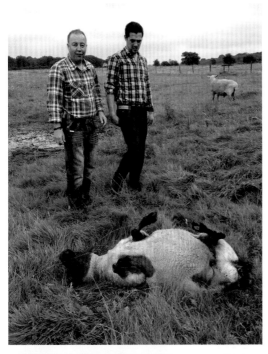

Adrian McHugh and Nicholas Millward saving the sheep!!

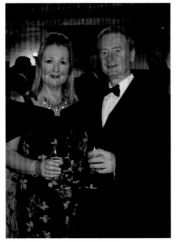

Linda Millward and Nick Woodall.

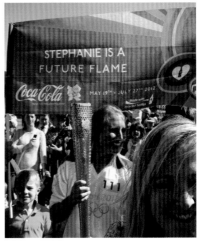

Stephanie carrying the Olympic Torch.

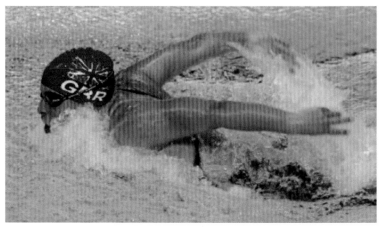

Stephanie swimming butterfly.

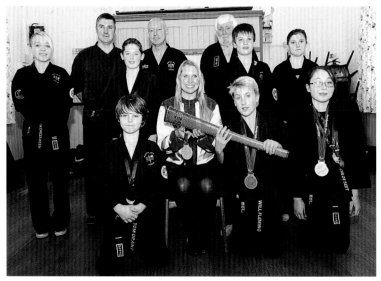

*Martial Arts Leisure – Tom Grant Black belt grading 3rd November 2013
Stephanie centre. Tom Grant front row left. Photo back row from L-R
Georgia Keen, Dave, Nick Bevan (Sensei), Mike. Middle row from L-R
Tom Donnelly, Thomas Stevens, Tammy. Front row from L-R Tom Grant,
Stephanie Millward, Will Flemming and Chloe.*

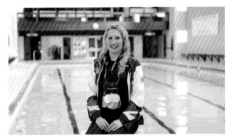

Stephanie at Springfield leisure centre the home of Corsham Swimming club.

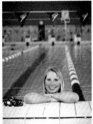

Stephanie in one of her favourite places!!

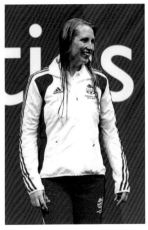

Stephanie at Commonwealth Games 2010 in Delhi, India.

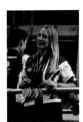

Stephanie on bus tour around London after the London 2012 Paralympics.

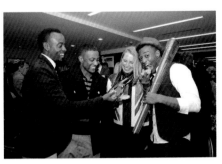

Stephanie with JLS having fun!!

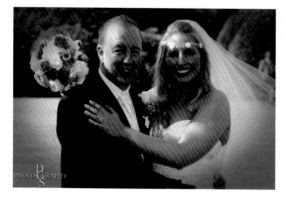

Stephanie and Adrian McHugh on their wedding day 04.05.2013.

Stephanie with her mum and dad (Linda and Mike Millward) on Stephanie's wedding day.

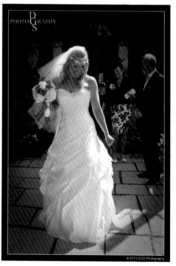

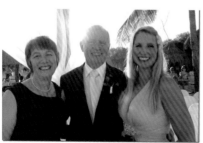

Diana and Mike Millward with Stephanie.

without paying me back. It wasn't a small sum with the total being thousands of pounds. I had trusted my apparent friends but they say you are meant to keep enemies closer possibly so that they don't get away with their bad deeds. My mum organised for me to take them to court to try to get the money back and after weeks of getting worried about the money they were forced to pay it back, slowly but surely. These friends were obviously not the type that anyone wants. With Adrian, all he did was the opposite. He gave me presents all the time: a smile, a hug, chocolates, cards, CDs or books. He just kept giving.

Adrian had played football professionally for Bristol City football club before they ran out of money and had to sign off a number of players, Adrian being one of them. He had always dreamed of playing football in a top team with other top football players. His dream was forced to die and I often feel that I am rubbing his nose in it. I have reached my dream but unfortunately he will never reach his. I hope that maybe indirectly I am helping him through my success.

When Adrian saw me swimming he said that he was impressed with my pretty strokes and that I should start training again. Since this time he has been a huge support, always by my side, always catching me when I fall and always cheering me on when I swim my races. When Adrian asked me to marry him it seemed the most perfect thing and the word Yes came out of my mouth as if I had said it a hundred times before. It was meant to happen. I was meant to be with my angel. I was meant to look after Adrian and for him to look after me. Adrian is that Ken I had often dreamed about and finally I play the role of Barbie, the perfect girl with the perfect life!

Adrian, please can you inject yourself just so that I can be certain you know how I feel every two days? Please can you do this terrible thing that I have been forced to do? Please show me you can be there for me always when I need your strength by my side and your arms holding me close. Please show me you know how strong I have been with the needles and please take some of my pain away. He stuck the needle in knowing that this would motivate me to keep on going. It was the right thing to do and Adrian shone after knowing that he could do anything if he needed to. I watched in amazement that someone would do something so unnecessary just to show me how much they cared about me. My heart swelled and the deep warmth in my body made me smile. This terrible deed I had to put myself through was no longer something I had to do on my own, Adrian and my mum were there for me every time even if it was often only in my mind.

Now I have my goals and I know what I want to do in life. Adrian has brought all my dreams alive and hopefully I can, and will, bring his dreams alive too. Adrian has made me so happy that even the MS doesn't matter anymore. Together, we are planning for a stunning wedding, a nice house and a lovely family.

A perfect life for my perfect world!

CHAPTER 47

Patients Advisory Board

I prayed and I begged and I hoped, and eventually a little bit of good luck came my way! I was very lucky and a large drug company asked me to be a part of their Patients Advisory Board! Being a part of the PAB included travelling to exotic locations, giving my opinion on the injections I was giving myself and their ease of use, and enjoying the lovely company of other PAB members, none of whom were English!

This all started in 2004 when I was asked to attend an MS seminar in Birmingham. A friend of mine agreed to drive me there and we had a lovely time with people recognising me either as the swimmer who got MS or the girl from the House of Commons; either was great! While I was in Birmingham a young lady asked me if I would like to be a part of the PAB and I obviously agreed. The first trip I went to as part of the board was to Berlin, the home of MS. This is where the founders of Betaferon had their main buildings. On this trip we were taken around the drug company's offices and we saw in great detail what the drug companies were working on. It was amazing to think the cures for all the illnesses starts here! We were given stunning five star hotels to stay in and the meals we were given were fantastic! I felt like a real part of the group when I had to stand up and say who I was and which country I was representing! 'Stephanie Millward, Great Britain, had MS since 1999, age seventeen.'

Everyone on the trip was lovely and I was allowed to take another person with me as my company for the trips and on this occasion I took my mum. We had a great time enjoying everything that was given to us and we gave all of our opinions on the drugs. I felt special being given this opportunity!

A year later I received some paperwork asking me to go to Prague and be a part of the PAB again! Wow! Who can I take with me? Kristy seemed the perfect choice and she agreed straight away! We had a fantastic time and on the last night we got so drunk that we were unable to go on the tour on the last day because we were so ill! In 2006 Kristy came with me again but this time it was to Rome! Both Prague and Rome were stunning places but the road sense was horrendous and the pedestrian crossings were completely ignored, wheelchair or no wheelchair! Rome was awe-inspiring and on our last night Kristy and I remembered the year before and controlled the drink! We ate a lovely meal inside an aquarium which was wonderful, with sharks and other large fish swimming over and around us!

In 2007 Adrian came with me to Barcelona. We had a wonderful time and we both enjoyed meeting all the PAB members again. Adrian was completely amazed with the hotel that we stayed in as there was a swimming pool on the roof! We were again amazed by the food that was offered to us. On one occasion we were taken to the famous café Els Quatre Gats (The Four Cats) where Picasso had eaten with his arty friends! Wow! We were given huge lobsters, squid, prawns, haddocks, cod and oysters! A wonderful array of fish in a five star restaurant!

I was planning to finish taking Betaferon in 2007 or 2008 and so I knew I had to inform the drugs company that I could no longer be a part of the PAB. This I felt was a real shame as I had made some good friends on the PAB and I had enjoyed the events thoroughly! On my last trip in Berlin I told everyone I was intending to start swimming again and that I would have to come off the drug and this would mean that I would have to get out of the PAB. Everyone was upset because I wasn't going to be seeing them again and worried for me if coming off the drugs didn't work for me. But they also were very strong for me and wished me good luck with the swimming, each of them saying that they could never do what I was thinking of doing and that they found me very inspiring!

Inspiring? I did wonder what they meant by this. How can someone who quits using the drugs that they found helped them at least for the first three years when they went from being completely paralysed and struggled to walk, to being on their feet and learning to stand, be inspiring? Now they are looking to stay well without drugs and moving to the pool where they can count on the water to keep them up. I am not sure 'inspiring' is the word. I had been giving myself injections for eight years when I stopped them and now I was giving up on them hoping that exercise and bringing my dream back to life would make me better. Inspiring? Headstrong and a little bit foolish I would say.

'At least Stephanie won't need to worry about walking,' I heard someone say! No, you are right. Walking won't be important as I will be a swimmer again! Can I realise my Olympic dreams as a Paralympian? Would it be the same as swimming as an able-bodied person?

Thank you, Betaferon, for giving me back my spark for life and thank you, PAB, for taking me to some wonderful places and for giving me a reason to like the MS! I feel that sometimes we meet people for a reason and the Patients Advisory Board was a wonderful reason and everything on this occasion turned out perfectly. The Patients Advisory Board was a definite good thing in among all those bad ones!

CHAPTER 48

Holidays!

Adrian and I spent our first Valentines' day in style, riding on a gondola in Venice and then joining in all the celebrations. We stayed in a hotel in St Mark's Square which is located in the centre of Venice. This is where all the celebrities come for the famous Valentines' day celebrations. Everybody dresses up in very decorative costumes with matching masks. These celebrations last for the whole week and Adrian and I were amazed at both the costumes and the atmosphere. It was a wonderful experience! We also went to see the usual landmarks and saw loads of places on the gondola trip. The whole holiday was fantastic and I would recommend it to anyone!

After our first holiday we got the bug and had to go again. This time we went to Marmaris, Turkey which proved a bit of a disappointment. We paid to go all-inclusive but this seemed just a good reason to eat and drink even if you didn't need it. We have decided to stay away from all-inclusive for the future. The hotel we stayed in was very nice but the swimming pool was freezing and so I couldn't even get my toes in. I was annoyed that I couldn't swim and a little fed up that the pool wasn't up to scratch.

We went on two trips; the first was to the natural hot springs in the mountains where apparently Cleopatra bathed. Amazingly, we were allowed to swim in these hot springs and so we did! I especially enjoyed this trip because I bought a bright pink bikini and Adrian bought a stunning marble chess set. The second trip was to some natural mud baths! It took us five hours in a hot bus to get there but it was worth the trip! After caking his body in mud Adrian then had to force himself to stand under a freezing cold shower to clean the mud off. I had stayed in the sun sunbathing so I just laughed at his obvious distress which infuriated him but made us both laugh more! On the way back from the mud baths we were taken on a slight detour to a carpet factory where we watched as people made the carpets. I was enthralled at how they made these fantastic carpets and had to buy one. When I was in Jeddah, my family had some handmade carpets similar to these handmade ones and so I felt obliged to buy one. I felt drawn to the carpets and the good memories linked to my childhood in Jeddah - I wanted to bring one back for old time's sake. The carpet I bought was going to be shipped to my front door and to make sure it was the same carpet I had signed the back of it in Turkey! To my mum's amazement, when it arrived at my front door it was the same carpet I had fallen for!

My next holiday was with my mum to Columbus, Ohio, America to stay with Kristy who had been offered the dream job working as a fashion designer for a large company! This was a wonderful trip and I got to drive a Mustang! My mum and I had a bit of an embarrassing day when she was being mean to some guys who were parked in our way meaning that we couldn't get out of the drive. Mum went and spoke to them and then we went to the car anxious to get going. We burst out laughing when mum tried to drive the car. We were sitting in the wrong seats and mum was in the right side of the car which in America is a passenger seat. Hysterical laughter lasted for about five minutes before we swapped seats and eventually moved the car!

While Kristy was working and we were driving her car around Ohio we went the wrong way on the motorway about three times, went down a one way street completely the wrong way and generally had a great time. The shopping was fantastic and the restaurants were brilliant as they kept refilling your drinks and were very courteous and well-mannered. I loved Ohio and can't wait to go back. Kristy is so lucky.

The next holiday was to Luxor, Egypt. Adrian and I had a marvellous time here flying on hot air balloons over the Valley of the Kings as well as seeing Tutankhamen's tomb! Our four star hotel was very nice and we met a couple who had been involved in swimming before. This former swimming coach had noticed my good strokes and had assumed I was a swimmer. After approaching me I told him my story about getting MS and that I was thinking about coming back into swimming but was still a little unsure. This coach, and another Scottish coach who was on the same holida,y both tried to convince me to start training properly again. The seeds were sown and I started training as soon as I got home. The sites in Egypt were amazing and the heat was immense. We both came back a lovely colour from a holiday we loved.

Barcelona, as part of the Patients Advisory Board, was the next holiday. Five stars all the way Adrian and I felt privileged. We were given lobsters, duck, beef, steak and prawns at incredible restaurants such as the Three Cats as well as in the hotel. We loved walking down the Ramblas and even doing the work for the PAB was very enjoyable. What a wonderful occasion! This is the only hotel I have ever seen with a swimming pool on the roof! Wow!

Christmas came and went and the next holiday arrived with huge smiles. The Caribbean! Adrian had seen the holiday in the travel agents close to where he lived and had known that this would be the perfect place for us. Antigua for two weeks in a good hotel with its pools, the sea, sand and the 20/20 cricket! I had started training before this holiday and Adrian saw this as a wonderful warm weather training facility! I got up early to swim a session then lay in the sun all day enjoying myself before doing another session in the afternoon.

Adrian and I met a young lady in one of the sun cream shops. Lucrethia was fantastic for us as she informed us of the best creams, of the best sites and she told us about the 20/20 cricket match that she was getting tickets for. As I struggled with her name I nicknamed Lucretia 'Lucky', which she enjoyed. Lucky bought us tickets for the 20/20 match and we went as a group. As she was a local we were able to sneak in everywhere! In among a large number of spectators we cheered for the teams with our score cards. On one side of the card was the number four and on the other was the number six. The atmosphere was electric. We were told that only the rich people stood in the stands and that everyone else sat on the grass. Everyone was so friendly and it was a carnival atmosphere. The cricket was good and I cheered for both teams ignorant of which side I was sat on. Somebody next to us pointed to Sir Viv Richards who was walking towards us. We ran to say hi and to get an autograph!! I kissed Sir Viv's cheek and gave him a hug! I felt very lucky! We also spotted another of Adrian's heroes - a very tall Cuertly Ambrose! We didn't get to speak to him but were thrilled that we had seen him! This was a wonderful event and it makes both Adrian and I smile to think about the fantastic day! Thank you, Lucky!

We took a day trip of a lifetime to Barbuda which has white sand and lovely blue sea but the problem lies with getting there. We had to ride on a catamaran in a very rough sea for a full hour and a half. It would have been fine without the sound of people throwing up and screaming and crying, all adding to the sound of the boat crashing against the waves. Adrian was holding me in place trying not to get thrown over the side of the boat. Our hands were very sore afterwards and when the boat finally pulled into the shore the relief was incredible. 'Is there another way back?' we all asked. The answer was 'No, just the way we had come. 'Oh no!

The day was an experience which was good but we are certain we will not go back! The white sand and the blue sea do not beat that awful journey. Going back, the journey was better as the driver of the catamaran tried to ride the waves causing less bumps and less sickness. Climbing into bed that night we felt exhausted and relieved! Our best trip of the fortnight was a guided tour around the island of Antigua. We were shown many plants that do the job of plasters, saw famous dock yards, saw other sites and bought some handmade jam! We travelled around the whole island in one day and saw some breath-taking scenery. Kissing Lucky goodbye we felt sadness and promised her that we would be back eventually. Lucky has added me as a friend on Facebook so we can stay in touch even if Adrian and I

CHAPTER 49
Beijing Paralympic Trials 2008

I came back from Egypt with stars in my eyes, deciding I would definitely get back into swimming properly. The Beijing Olympic trials are just round the corner: what should I do to get fit for this competition? A coach would be useful as plodding up and down at the Springfield Centre swimming pool in Corsham every couple of mornings isn't going to be good enough. When I worked in Trowbridge the company, DC Leisure, had sponsored me by allowing me the use of the swimming pool for free at Trowbridge sports centre. I felt so honoured by this so maybe they could help?

Adrian and I got on the British Swimming website to try to find out some information and to get contacts and in the end we spotted Stephen Fivash who lived in Melksham, which was pretty close by. We sent him an email and asked to meet up with him which we did at Springfield Centre Corsham! I was very nervous when the day came to meet Steve and the fluttering in my stomach made me feel a little sick.

Steve was very sweet and he made us feel at ease straight away. I got into the pool to show him a few of my strokes and he commented straight away on my backstroke. He said 'You might not be fit enough yet to do two hundreds or one hundreds but we can definitely try you on that 50m Backstroke! Steve took a few times for some of the lengths I did and you could see he was excited with the splits! After the session he confirmed that I had a new coach for my goal to get to London 2012! I was very pleased with myself - everything was great! I did a few hard weeks with Steve making a few tweaks to my strokes. My dreams were alive. Just imagine if I could just pick up my gold medals! I am almost there I could be good again!

As we know it's not that easy and especially for me where everything seems to go wrong if there is a chance. Weeks had gone by and the training was going well and then Steve said something that shocked me: 'I have put you in for a race in Sheffield.'

'What? I have just started I don't want to race yet.' I wasn't sure that I was ready to race or ready to get another failure.

'You'll be fine.'

Okay, can I really do this after all these years? What will it be like? Will it be the same as it was before, before I got sick? Can I beat my personal bests (PBs)? So many things were going through my mind that before I knew it I was by the pool side at Ponds Forge in Sheffield surrounded by loads of disabled people. Everyone kept saying 'Hi Stephanie' and a lot of people seemed to know who I was even though I didn't know anything about them. It was such a strange feeling. It was almost as though they had been waiting for me to turn up since I had been diagnosed almost ten years ago!

I was swimming in a national competition for the South West against all the other regions. I was selected to swim 100m Backstroke. Going up to the race I was terrified and it all felt so different to how I had remembered. The swim was horrible. The time was horrible. I got out crying. It hurt so much to see the times on the board. My 1:05.18 personal best was replaced by the awful time of 1:18.56 What am I doing? I burst out crying again. It was awful. I cried looking around for Adrian. Why am I doing this to myself? I have MS. I am sick now. I shouldn't be swimming. Adrian found me and put his arms around me.

'Well done you won your race. It was close, but you won!'

'No I lost! I lost it all!' I remembered all that time training I had spent at Bath University and all those fast times I had swam.

'Let's go home, let's get out of here,' I said, and four hours later we were back, back to the place of safety where no one was looking at me and where no one was putting a label on me. I was safe. It had felt so foreign on the poolside trying to swim fast again. Why did I do that to myself? I know why, I want to win that Olympic gold medal that I was supposed to have won all those years ago!

A few weeks passed and, again, Steve said there was another race again in Sheffield but it was the Nationals for disability swimmers and that this was where I needed to be classified to see which group or classification I should be swimming in. I said yes again even though I remembered all those horrible thoughts and feelings from last time. This time I would know what to expect. Now I can swim fast like I did all those years ago as I have done more training so I will be so much faster!

I was again by the side of the pool at Ponds Forge Sheffield with disabled people all around me: limbs on the floor, children with one arm, one leg and wheelchairs everywhere. Many smiling, happy faces of people so happy to be there competing who wanted to swim to show off what they could do even with a disability! They all wanted to be here!

I felt like I was in the wrong place again. I have two legs and two arms so I didn't have a disability. The classification went quite well with the classifiers asking me to do all sorts of manoeuvres from standing on one leg, which proved difficult, to swinging my arms around so they could see how coordinated I was. The classification finished and I felt exhausted! I was awarded the S10 classification which is the most able class! S1 to S10 are physically disabled swimmers and S11 to S13 are eyesight disabilities. S14 is where the swimmer has special needs. Back to the physical classifications, S1 are very disabled swimmers and S10 are the most able missing one thing or limb. A swimmer classified as S9 would be missing two limbs or two things like balance and coordination and swimmer classified as S8 would be missing three things. I felt quite proud that I was an S10 and therefore basically very able.

In a flash my race was next. I was helped to the blocks, the gun fired and I was away. Backstroke, my event, my race.

As I turned for the last fifty metres of the one hundred metre race I felt so tired and weak. I was slowing and my body was hurting. It wasn't not like this in training! Then I touch the wall. What was my time? Did I break the world record? My PB, was that smashed? No! Look at that time 1.16. Oh my gosh, I can't swim anymore. It's all gone, the only thing I have left in this world. My swimming has gone forever. The MS has ruined everything.

The tears started before I even tried to get out of the pool and then when I struggled to get out Adrian had to start helping to pull me out. My body couldn't stop crying, my dream was over in my eyes for the second time in one life. Why am I bothering? Why did I believe I could come back after all those awful years? My life was never going to be easy especially with this rotten illness but dreams live forever and can never be broken: why did my dream have to be torn from me yet again? This is so cruel.

I tried to stop crying and Adrian told me that I won the race and that the girl I beaten had not lost a race in two years! She was the GB number one and I had just beaten her!

'You are Great Britain's number one swimmer for 100m Backstroke in the S10 category. That's great Stephanie! You have qualified for Beijing 2008.'

'No, it's not. Look at that time! I could swim that time when I was twelve.'

'Stephanie, you are a different swimmer now. We have to build back up to get to that level again. You can do it, it is going to take a long time with lots of hours back in the pool, but the speed is there. You just have to believe in your body and believe in yourself! You can beat that time of 1.05.18 you swam as a 15/16 year old but it will take time'.

I know he's right, I am so frustrated with myself and with the MS.
I know I can beat my old time.
I need all my little things in place to do it.
Eyes dry and on our way back home to tell my mum.
Better not tell her what the time was though as she would feel the pain too.

I was now the fastest S10 100m Backstroke female swimmer and would therefore represent Great Britain as part of the Paralympics in Beijing, I needed to get an international classification as well as my original classification which was just a national classification. I was therefore invited to go to the Denmark Open Meet 2008 where I could get my international classification!

This was my first open meet competing for Great Britain as part of their Paralympic team. It was so strange coming back to racing for GB and being part of the national team again – kind of. I wasn't sure if it felt the same as when I was younger and swam for the able-bodied team. It was always so exciting to pack my bag ready for the trip and to meet the team members. On this occasion I was a bit anxious and worried about what it would be like among all the swimmers with a disability. I have never had an issue with disabilities as when I was younger I was close friends with Mandy who only had one leg. I had never understood why people acted differently to people with a disability when really they are still just the same as anybody else but with an extra thing to think about. I had nothing to worry about as we had already competed together at the National competitions in Sheffield to qualify for this event. It was so exciting being dropped off at the airport and although we were in our own clothes and not the GB kit, as we had done every time we competed as an able-bodied GB athlete, it was still wonderful to meet some of the other swimmers. The flight was good as I love travelling by air and it always makes me think about holidays and flying to nice places!

While I was in Denmark racing I had to be reclassified by an international classifier so that I could compete in countries outside of the UK. Every Paralympic swimmer needs this re-classification. After my original classification I was awarded an S10 classification but after this re-classification I was moved to an S9 which meant that I was now more disabled than I had been at the first classification. When I heard about this new classification I cried and cried and felt so depressed. Although it was embarrassing to cry in front of everyone it showed them all, myself included, that I had a fear about the MS and about getting worse. Dropping to a lower class meant that I was more disabled than I was before, it was proof that I was getting worse. How do I stop this progression of the illness? I met the guy who reclassified me a few years later and I told him how annoyed I had been! He just smiled! Truthfully, after the initial upset I came to terms with being an S9 classification. I had a better and more confident feeling about this so I can now swim well as an S9. Beijing Paralympic Games here I come!

Steve Fivash was a great coach but wasn't allowed to be my coach because of his role as part of British Swimming so I therefore had to find another one. I went to Bath Uni to see if I could train there; the university coach watched me swim a session and said that I would never be a good enough swimmer to train with him! 'She will never be a good enough swimmer!' he had said but I believed otherwise! I bet he felt a bit stupid when Bath Uni put the huge congratulations banner up in the Bath University sports training village after I had swam well at the World Championships 2013 winning four gold World Championships medals!

I remembered all my amazing coaches when I was younger, Peggy Tanner and Julia Airlie at Corsham ASC with Sylvia Howland helping as a great support! David Lyles and then Ian Turner at Bath University, Steve Fivash, Cherie Baker, Dave Pegg at Melksham ASC who was lovely and the amazing Bernie Nichols who was a wonderful man. Little did I know that my next coach was going to be an incredible help for my career and for my dream!

CHAPTER 50
Swimming with the Stars! June 2008

Swimming and coaching in Corsham, Trowbridge, Melksham and Bath was good and I enjoyed all of it but when Adrian took me to my friend Sonia Bush's house for a meeting, I knew that something wonderful was about to happen. We sat down with a cup of tea and Colin Bush, the ex-coach of the successful Chippenham Town football club, chaired the meeting. He started off by talking about motivation and asked me about what I wanted to do with the swimming. I still had the strokes, I was still very good and I could be the best in the world and all we needed was the correct coaching to readjust the effects of a ten-year break from swimming and to get me fit. Colin went through the options: I could remain at Corsham ASC travelling miles to each of the pools fitting in my swims around my work, trying to find the pool time available around my forty-hour working week, or I could move to Swansea. Swansea? Swansea was a million miles away.

Colin and Sonia told me that in Swansea I would have a wonderful coach and be with swimmers of my ability and that I would be able to realise all my dreams. They were very inspiring as they had been since I first met them while still very sick. They convinced me totally that even though I had to leave my home, my boyfriend, my mum, my dog and my friends it would be worth it in the end. There were no available spaces at my home club in Bath because I was disabled. I was very excited about the move to Wales. Billy Pye, the coach for the disability squad in Swansea, had arranged originally for me to stay in a bed and breakfast with a lovely couple called Richard and Merle James who were very sweet. I paid them the forty pounds per night and they treated me as a daughter. They were very friendly and incredibly kind.

Billy arranged for me to move into a house owned by Wales Swimming and told me that the coach who normally stays there had agreed that I should stay there for free for the seven weeks prior to the Paralympics. Wow! Everything seemed so easy and so well planned as though this was the only option available because it was so well organised. I didn't think about how much it would cost me eventually or whether I was going to swim in Wales after Beijing 2008. I didn't question whether I was staying or going. It was already written in the stars! I was meant to be swimming in Swansea. I was meant to be swimming with the stars!

The move went well and the training was very hard but I loved every minute. I called Adrian many times a day telling him about the sessions and about the swimmers at Swansea and about Billy who seemed to have a telepathic instinct and knew exactly what I needed. I missed everybody but the determination to be the best was strong and I was excited about the prospect of being the swimmer from 1998 again, before I got sick. Just imagine if I beat those times! Just imagine if I get a lifetime personal best! I was realising my dreams; I was going to the Olympic Games!

My main training partner, Dave Roberts, hads been doing it for twelve years, got the CBE, got the medals; he had done it all before. Dave is an interesting individual who seems to know everything about different sports and he discusses these with Billy on many occasions. Dave was very confident and I grew strong because of this confidence when I first came over to the Swansea Performance centre. He knows exactly what he is doing and he knows he is the best at what he does. He would call out the start time for me even if he swam in on the last second. This helps as when I swim hard my eyesight gets worse and I suffer with my eyes jumping back and forth, up and down and I struggle to see the clock. Dave called out the times: 'Five seconds, four, three, two, one.' This was much needed and I learned to almost rely on it. I thought of Dave as a big soft cuddly toy. If I needed a friend, he would be a friend. If I needed a pound for the lockers, he would lend me a pound. If I needed to discuss swimming competitions, he would know the date, the location and the time. He was very organised and whenever I struggled with memory problems Dave was the answer to my prayers!

Also training at the same time as me and Dave were Ellie Simmonds, Matt Whorwood, Liz Johnson, Gareth Duke, Ant Stephens, Jenny Coughlin and Graham Edmunds. Each has a disability of their own and each has a story that would amaze millions.

Gareth Duke is quite a remarkable person. Due to complications with his kidneys he has to undergo dialysis treatment three times a week. Whenever I see Gareth he always smiles and is so extremely positive about his life and about his swimming. Having had six months off for medical treatments, Gareth came back with more vigour and fight than I have seen in anyone else. His strive to be as good as possible remains apparent and daily he has to act twice his age. He has to consider things that he is far too young to consider. He is an incredible person and I hope he always remains well.

Graham Edmunds has been a definite help for me because of his extremely positive and motivational attitude to life. If you are feeling sorry for yourself you just need to say Hi to Gra' and he will make you smile again. I respected his help immensely and I hope to stay his friend for a long time, and I am certain that anyone who has ever met Graham will long for his friendship and his strength. When I am swimming a very hard threshold or heart rate set, Graham will see me struggling and will give me some comforting words making me strive for faster times and for better consistency. He is a thoughtful person and with the strength that he conveys is very powerful. I long to have his confidence and sure footed approach to life and when he voices his opinion the words are usually inspiring. On many occasions when Graham sees me struggling he will swim next to me to try to get the fight back in me to keep going. This is something I will be forever thankful for.

When I win medals it will be partially down to Graham for the inspiration, partially down to Dave for calling out the times and for his excellence in his sport, partially down to Gareth for his strength and determination and very much down to Billy, my wonderful coach.

Billy is fantastic. He knows everything about swimming and everything about swimming fast. I ask him the smallest question and he will give me a forty page documentary about why we do that and how this will help that and how it will help the stroke and why it has that effect. Billy looked up every aspect of my illness, Multiple Sclerosis, before he met me and he knew that I could have balance problems, eyesight problems, spasticity or speech problems. He had looked for anything that might go wrong. He knew about my illness probably better than me. When I first met Billy he seemed like a very strong young man with the whole world in his hands. He was very determined to make me who I wanted to be. He is inspiration in itself as he can make anyone good. He can see the mistakes instantly and he has cunning ways to correct them. Billy said straight away how good my strokes were and he asked me how fast I used to swim: 1.05.18 for 100m Backstroke when I was fifteen.

Billy listened to the copies of my songs and he watched the DVD that Stephen Brown had created for me about my fight with MS and my desire to be the best in the pool. Billy was interested in my life, in my fight, in everything I have been through with the MS. I felt important, as though the self-confidence I had lost so severely while aged only seventeen could start rebuilding itself again. Billy is someone I look to for advice and strength and anything I don't get from Adrian or from my mum or from any of the other swimmers. Swimming here in Swansea I feel complete, as though I had to go through all that pain to get this wonderful thing at the end. Like childbirth, I suppose. The mother has to go through all that pain but they get the wonderful baby at the end. The pain is almost worth it. In my life swimming with the stars and being loved by Adrian and my family and friends makes my pain worth it.

As part of the Great Britain team I was monitored quite a lot more and I had to produce a spreadsheet every week which I then had to send to a select number of staff members. The spreadsheet contained my swim session plans and total metreage and it told of details about my strength and conditioning (S&C) sessions. At the bottom of the spreadsheet it had details about any races I had recently swam and I had to record my times and whether they were a PB time or not. These spreadsheets (log sheets) were a useful way of seeing how far I swam every week and if I wanted to see which sessions I swam just before I raced an amazing time: it is a simple way of checking!

I also had to complete a different form of spreadsheet for drug testing where I had to select one hour out of every single day that I must be available for drug testing. Most athletes use one of their training sessions as this hour as it is an easy location to record. I often use my swim sessions as my drug-testing slot. If I am not swimming on a certain day I have to select an easy time in a simple location, for example dinner time at my home, when I know I will not be snoozing and therefore have the chance of missing the door bell and getting a missed test. We are only allowed two missed tests which is when the drug tester turns up at your slot but you for whatever reason are not there. The third time will mean a ban. In return for completing these spreadsheets I am offered some money from UK Sport and the National Lottery. This funding is called the APA (Athlete Personal Award). UK Sport distributes Lottery funding through the World Class Performance Programme to help our best and most talented athletes achieve podium success at the Olympic and Paralympic Games. Athletes are nominated for support by the governing body of their sport. This is a contribution to the living and personal sporting costs incurred while training and competing as an elite athlete. The APA application process is managed by UK Sport. Nominated athletes receive an application form which must be completed in full and returned promptly. An offer letter will then be sent out if you qualify for an award. The exact amount of the APA will vary depending on your performance category and any other income you receive. Each APA is offered for a maximum of twelve months. If you are nominated again at the end of an award period, you will need to complete a new application form.

Completing the spreadsheets and receiving my APA is such an exciting reminder that I am part of the Great Britain swimming team! I am part of the GBR swimming team and training with the stars. I am doing what I want to do and I am doing it even though I have MS!

CHAPTER 51

China (again!) –
The Paralympics

A dream? A hope? I am less certain now. I had expected a lot from the Olympic and the Paralympic Games but the dream experience had not been quite as I had expected. I suppose it all arrived too early. The life I had desired seemed somewhat nullified. A disappointment maybe, but a number of useful things were learned from this event which can only help me on my way to that dream gold medal.

The Paralympics were going to be held in Beijing, China. Ten years after my first introduction to China in Shanghai I was returning to the place where I competed last before the MS began. What am I feeling? Nerves? I was absolutely scared stiff. Why was I being forced to go back? Was this a way for me to get over the demons that I had had since getting the MS or was it a way of rubbing my nose in it? Shanghai had been a wonderful trip except for the swimming part, which was laden down with MS and regret. China had therefore been a good experience for me but it has always been linked to swimming badly and therefore not doing what I was meant to do. It happened again.

The Paralympics were a huge disappointment for me and right from the start everything went wrong. Maybe I should have foreseen what was going to happen. Here is a list of the reasons I believe I didn't swim as well in Beijing as I would have liked, other than the obvious psychological fact that it was in China!

1. Not enough training

I think that the seven/eight weeks while being coached by Billy were fantastic, but there was no way I should have believed that I was ready to swim my best ever races having had such a small amount of training. I didn't have the stamina to keep going as was proven in all my races. I hit 75m very much ahead of the field but then fatigue played its part and the small amount of training did not give me the extra energy I needed to finish the races.

2. Incorrect coach

The weeks of training with Billy would have finished nicely with a correct taper but instead I was awarded a different coach to work with when we went to the holding camp in Macau (and then onto Beijing) who worked mainly on distance for each session. If I had been allowed to have my own coach training me in Beijing I believe it would have been an easier fight for me but instead I was stressed from having to change coaches and then having to get used to this new coach before even starting to think about why we were in Beijing. I think this was a major player in me swimming badly, or at least not up to my own high standards.

3. Routine

I work off routines. I tell my mind what is happening and generally my body follows what it is being told to do. If anything changes or goes off routine then the body gets confused and does not do what it is meant to do. It has taken me almost ten years to understand my body and I don't expect everyone else to just know what is right or wrong, but please just try to see it from my point of view. My body has been through stages of not moving correctly, of not being able to see, of having no bladder or bowel control, of being completely paralysed for quite long periods of time. Please just understand that allowing me to have my routines is a small price to pay, especially when it is me paying it every single day.

4. Other swimmers
Other swimmers did a few very annoying things such as picking Speedo signs off costumes while I was trying to sleep. This was especially annoying on nights before I was swimming and they weren't due to swim. I have learned now to room with someone who will swim on the same days as me or at least choose someone who will understand that I need to sleep in preparation for a race.

5. On my feet all the time
I was told on a number of occasions to get off my feet. This was probably a good thing because it made me sit down but, incidentally, I never use a wheelchair and am always on my feet so I doubt it would have made a difference!

6. Holding camp
We were taken to a holding camp in Macau for the week leading up to Beijing. I wasn't used to being away from home for that long. I missed my family and I especially missed Adrian. At the end of the trip to Macau I just wanted to fly home and not start my Paralympic debut. My dream was finished before it had even begun.

7. I didn't deserve to win it
I had not swam enough or worked hard enough. If I had won it would have been a joke and the whole Paralympics would have been a let-down. The fact that I didn't swim well let me know that the Paralympics is something you have to earn and thus need to work hard for. I had trained so hard to get to Sydney and I would have treasured the whole experience but with Beijing it came too early and I just wanted to go home. I wasn't ready to swim the races. I hadn't trained hard enough. In my eyes I didn't deserve to be there.

As you have just read, a lot of things didn't seem to be right. Everybody likes to invent an excuse to explain why they didn't perform but I honestly feel that these aren't excuses, just relevant reasons and a combination of breakdowns that played their part in my life on the journey to, and in, Beijing. Beijing had been everything a Paralympic

Games could have been with many picturesque features and wonderful scenes and sights and I felt proud to be there, but something felt wrong right from the start. When I met Adrian we had agreed to chase the Olympic/Paralympic dream in London 2012; Beijing just jumped in the way! I had felt that I wasn't ready for the event, that I didn't deserve to be there and so in some ways I should not have gone. Realistically, I was fast enough to be there but my heart just didn't feel it.

When you get an opportunity to go to somewhere as huge as the Olympics/Paralympics I took up the challenge with only limited training under my belt. From where I had come to where I was going, well, we all hope for that happy ending. Many members of my family spent their money to support my races. They wanted me to swim well even though they perhaps didn't believe I could, not yet. I have since realised that for a huge amount of people the achievement I have gained was a huge dream come true and one which will stay with me for the rest of my life. I am now and always will be an Olympic/Paralympic swimmer which is something absolutely anyone would be proud of. In Beijing I came 4th, 5th and 6th in the whole wide world! Definitely not something to be upset about especially after only seven weeks of proper training!

London 2012 Paralympic Games, here I come!!

CHAPTER 52

Great Wall of China – Proposal!

'No, you are not allowed to go to the wall today. You need to support your team.'

What? I only wanted to go when the other swimmers were swimming their heats. Nobody needs the support for the heats; they are a bit of a waste of my time. I will be back for the finals. Surely they will never notice and anyway the cheering is really only needed from me for the finals.

They didn't notice! Thankfully!

I walked out of the Olympic Village like a thief trying to make sure that no one saw me sneak out, and made my way down the road where I could see the taxi waiting for me. The taxi was full of the rest of my family with Mister (Nicholas) being the only one who could not make it to Beijing. We set off to the Great Wall, one of the Great Wonders of the World. I could not wait and I was so excited, we all were. The chatting was incredible as we drove up to the queue for entry to the wall.

Adrian clasped my hand and we walked together to the queue. Kristy started giggling as she pulled Paul's sun hat over his eyes! This caused an inevitable play fight which amused us all. We went into the site and walked on top of the Wall peering over the edge, feeling our stomachs turn at the sheer height. Paul's phone started ringing as he was still at work, really, and so he dropped back discussing deals of his trade - trust Paul to work all the time!

Adrian seemed a little edgy and asked a few times what Paul was doing.

'Work,' I said. 'He has to make money somehow.'

Adrian always seems to carry huge bags around with him and I noticed he had his big bag with him today. Did he have a thermos of tea or has he brought lunch? I decided not to ask him!

Paul caught us up and it was here that Adrian grabbed his chance. He said later that his nerves were making him feel sick but he turned to me, stopping me in my path, knelt down on one knee and then, in front of the majority of my family he held out a sparkly white gold ring and asked me to marry him! I smiled holding the tears of exclamation away, and said 'Yes!' without even opening my mouth! How exciting! We are going to get married! We will be together forever! I won't be on my own. We can have kids, we can be happy!

Paul, Kristy and mum took loads of photos and we got given huge hugs and celebratory handshakes. I was still amazed and excited! Kristy said to me a little later that she knew he was going to ask me to marry him and in some ways I knew it too. It was just the right time and a perfect destination too which is something I mentioned when we first got together! ('Adrian, I would love for my husband to be to choose a perfect place to ask me to marry them, maybe while away on holiday in a sunny place with nice views.') I got exactly what I wanted - the Great Wall of China in September 2008 at the Paralympic Games. Adrian told me later that he had already asked my dad if he could have his permission to marry me! I think my mum wanted to be asked too as she was such a great support when the MS struck. Adrian and I asked my mum to be our wedding planner as I knew she would love that job!

There was only one issue on that day and that was how do we get down off this one thousand foot wall? The answer was to sit down on your bum and slide down a slide! Paul and Kristy excitedly flew down at one hundred miles per hour and then mum went at her speed which was closer to that of a snail; when I caught her up I had to put both feet down and stop while I waited for her to move a bit more. Adrian followed behind me and we started making up the queue. Oh, well. At least we enjoyed it!

Going back to the Paralympic village I had a smile plastered on my face and I wasn't surprised when people asked what the matter was. I showed off my ring and we discussed where I was going to get married. It didn't matter right then, I thought; it was an exciting thing to concentrate on later. None of the officials seemed to notice I had sneaked out or at least they didn't say anything. What a wonderful day - 14th September 2008, when Adrian proposed to me!

CHAPTER 53

Post-Paralympics, 2008

I had finally realised my dream of swimming at the Olympic/Paralympic Games but it didn't feel like it. I had originally wanted to swim in London 2012 Paralympics not Beijing. Beijing just got in the way. I had started with nothing, forty hours per week at work, three hours coaching in two different towns, Tai Kwon Do for two hours and travelling miles to get any pool time for myself. It was Bernie Nichols (my coach at this time) who introduced me to Steve Fivash. He told me how I could get funding. He lit the torch saying that there is funding available for swimmers who have met the criteria. I found it hard travelling to the pools and working full-time but I swam well in the national competition winning a number of races and gaining a qualifying time for Beijing. I had also won two European record times with my swims! It was here when I knew I could be the best in the world. My family was very pessimistic as they were very scared that I was going to get sick. Why can't they be strong when they know how hard I have already fallen? I needed their strength then more than they will ever know.

I wanted to get the funding and was offered it half-way through the year even though this is generally not allowed. Steve was told that he was not allowed to coach me so I had to find another coach. Cherie Baker was a 21-year-old girl who had a few years' experience coaching young club swimmers but probably didn't know how to train a disabled swimmer. Cherie worked hard coaching me for a while. I was swimming against professional swimmers and I was trying to swim as a part-time swimmer. I was taking big steps by trying to compete against them. I quickly proved that I was an able swimmer but I wanted the chance to race as well as I train. I wanted the funding. I woke up early every morning and stayed awake until at least eleven at night. I was trying to do everything. I did a lot of training at the weekend because that was when there was more pool time. I was training in public sessions so part of my time was spent overtaking members of the public.

The funding was good as it gave me an opportunity to stop working seven weeks prior to Beijing and to concentrate on the Paralympics that were fast approaching. Steve introduced me to Billy Pye over the phone and so I went to meet Billy in Swansea as this was where I could train full-time. Billy had 30 years' experience; he was at the top of the tree. He could definitely help me to reach my goals. Seven weeks of training before I went to the Paralympics. I had two European records and was new to funding. I trusted Billy to help me get what I wanted.

My funding was taken away from me after the Paralympics because of the bad swims. It is hard to take when the reason for me swimming badly was beyond my control. I enjoy stability and I was given a new coach for the Paralympics when I had just changed coaches anyway. I might have swam bad anyway but a few weeks later I won three world records, thereby proving that if the taper had been better and I had been with a coach that I trusted maybe I would have swam better in the Paralympics. These however are still maybes and we will never know for sure. The funding was be reduced. I had given up my job and moved countries (from England to Wales!) to realise my dream. The dream had not survived and here I was trying to pick up the pieces again. Why do people make it so difficult for me? Unfortunately, Beijing came a few weeks too early for me, bring on 2012.

I recorded my income and outgoings in a spreadsheet. I was losing £300 per month by being in Swansea. Although I had enough money at that moment, by losing that much per month I would soon be out of money. I was trying to represent my country but obviously this was impractical. I was living in a deficit. I ended up cutting down on the amount of food I bought as obviously rent and other bills were something I had to pay. Adrian often called me asking what I had eaten that day only to get the answer of some cereal or a banana because meat was far too expensive for me. Adrian knew I was struggling so he often brought food for me when he visited me on the weekends. I suppose that lack of excess cash helped me with my weight loss program! Before I got sick I was a very slender girl with no fat anywhere but when the MS arrived and I went suddenly from training ten two-hour sessions a week plus gym sessions and runs down to not being able to move so I piled the weight on. My clothes increased from size eight or ten up to eighteen! I was traumatised because I had worked so hard to eat correctly and do all the exercise I could. Even when I got sick I stayed eating almost nothing, worried that every mouthful was another size bigger in clothes. Billy Pye made me feel a bit better about my weight and he said with the training next year it would just drop off, which it did start to!

In a meeting I had with the people in charge of swimming I was asked whether I wanted to go to 2012? My answer was yes, but obviously if there was no funding available then no. I would not be able to go. I had realised my dream, I had been to the Paralympic Games. I should have felt happy but my desire was not satisfied as it had been messed up by an incorrect coach among other reasons. If everything had gone right I would have swam well at the Paralympics. I would have been a star as opposed to a depressed child trying to grow up. Maybe I should get over this dream and get on with reality. I had lived a difficult past ten years; why did I think it would change just because I had reached my goal? What a life!

Robert James was the wonderful guy who helped me sort out my funding problems. Robert was the accountant in charge of Swim Wales and was based at the pool where I trained. Robert offered me a part-time job in the accounts department which I loved. This gave me the ability to make up some of the debt that I was struggling with. Thanks Robert! I often tried to repay his friendship by driving him for a drink in the local Thai restaurant which I am certain we both enjoyed every trip. He is a wonderful person and has a heart of pure gold!

Coming back after the Beijing Paralympics was better than I had anticipated, even after winning no medals and getting only fourth, fifth and sixth place certificates. The media grabbed my story. Yeah, I hadn't done well at the Paralympics but I was always going for London 2012 anyway! The school where I went to for my GCSE and A-levels asked me to come and give a speech to them to try to inspire the children with my story. The Corsham Comprehensive School was the name of my school and it is also where my mum worked as a head teachers' secretary. I couldn't wait to do this speech and obviously the children were amazed with my story and the chance to meet an Olympian, or rather a Paralympian! This was a very special way to end Beijing 2008.

CHAPTER 54
Headteacher's Letter

Stephanie Millward
Chippenham
Wiltshire

24 October 2008

Dear Stephanie,

Thank you so much for being our guest of honour last night. Everybody thought you were wonderful. Your speech was so inspirational for the students, not to mention the adults! I hope you enjoyed it. As I mentioned, I will find the name of the student who took the photograph of Bath and arrange for them to sign it.

People were so thrilled to meet you that I am going to ask you if you wouldn't mind being our guest on two more evenings planned for later in the year. The first is Thursday 27 November at 19.30 when last year's year 11 will be awarded their GCSE certificates. The other evening is Tuesday 6 January, again at 19.30 when students will receive their A-level certificates.

The evenings are slightly smaller affairs. I do hope that you are available and would be willing to come.

Once again, many thanks for contributing to a wonderful evening and being such an inspiration to our students. I will never forget some of their faces when they actually shook the hand of an Olympic athlete.

Best wishes.

Yours sincerely,

Martin Williams
Headteacher

CHAPTER 55

Longmeadow Primary School

'Stephanie, I was wondering if you could do my wife Caroline a favour,' Mike Cox, the swimming friend who had asked me to teach Adrian how to swim, inquired during swimming at Corsham Springfield Centre one morning. Mike Cox did a lot of training as a triathlete and went on to compete in many Ironman competitions around the world.

'Yes, sure. What does she want me to do?'

'Caroline was wondering if you could visit her primary school and tell the children all about your life with swimming and about the Paralympics in Beijing.'

'Wow! Yeah, I would love to!' I confirmed.

I went to Longmeadow Primary School armed with items from the Paralympic Games and I was all dressed up in my GB tracksuit. The class welcomed me in with huge smiles! They had arranged a special Olympic seat for me to sit on and they had arranged Olympic badges all around their room. The place looked stunning!

I sat down on my allocated seat and a group of twenty enthusiastic children sat around me. They had organised themselves to ask questions and listen to my answers. I showed them a bag of medals I had already won and my mementos from Beijing. I adopted the school as my own and when I left I told them I would love to teach them how to swim and that I couldn't wait to see them again. What a wonderful day!

I was invited back to the school for a whole day with the children. They had organised a special breakfast and we sat and ate crumpets and toast and drank cups of tea. This was another perfect day at the school.

On my third visit back I taught the children how to swim. I had already spoken to Paul Parker from DC Leisure at Clarendon sports centre (the amazing company who had originally sponsored me and let me swim at the pool for free in the mornings) and he had said that we could have the hour at the pool for free which was lovely of them. All the children jumped in the pool and listened to my every word. A local paper called the *Wiltshire Times* took photos of us enjoying ourselves and our faces graced the paper the next day! After swimming we went back to the school and again had breakfast with cups of tea. On this occasion we also had pancakes because we had burned off so many calories! I again stayed all day loving the time I spent with the children.

I returned to this school many times and again after London to show them my medals! I feel attached to the school and love to see the smiles on their faces! Good luck everyone and thank you for everything, Caroline Cox, their amazing headteacher!

CHAPTER 56

BBC Sports Personality of the Year

Just after returning home from Beijing I received a letter inviting me to the BBC Sports Personality of the Year Awards. I felt privileged to get this invitation! I confirmed that I could go and then started looking for an outfit. Adrian had bought me a stunning black dress for my birthday so I decided this was the perfect choice. Dress, shoes, make-up! When I was getting dressed for this celebration I felt exactly the same as I did when I went to Corsham ASC's presentation evenings all those years ago. What would this event be like?

It was wonderful. I caught a taxi to the red carpet then went into the building. Everyone looked stunning. The venue was full of important people, the celebrities! Ellie Simmonds stayed close to me which was good because she recognised everyone so she kept telling me who they were. It was amazing to see all these really famous people! Ellie and I got loads of photos with them! It was unreal!

We were called to sit in our specific allocated seats. Mine was behind the legend Sir Bobby Charlton and Theo Walcot (football players!) and I was on the TV every time the camera went to Sir Bobby Charlton so they caught glimpses of me too! My mum and Adrian were watching on the TV and kept seeing me so I hope I was smiling.

The Beckham family were sitting in some of the front row seats and it was so weird but after a diversion on stage the Beckhams just disappeared and must have gone home without having to do any autographs or photos - clever!

I loved this BBC Sports Personality of the Year (SPOTY) and have enjoyed many other SPOTYs since. A lovely celebration of sporting expertise!

CHAPTER 57

My Future

I'm so proud of my past
But a little scared of the future
Find comfort in what I have done
Feel relief in how I am coping.

Amazement covers my face
The thrill of what I've achieved.
My family is worth a million pounds
Would I have coped without them?

Their love is never ending, their support is eternal
Their hopes and dreams are unstoppable!
The hurt inside, the pain
It's so hard to move on

The dreams that all have been broken
The memories that all have now gone
So proud of the past but that is now over
Have a blank page to fill and a new life to uncover.

CHAPTER 58

Meeting the Queen

Did I think I would ever meet the Queen? No, probably not. She is so important and so fantastic! Why would she want to meet me?

You have been invited to meet HRH the Queen in celebration of swimming for our country. Wow! I get to see the Queen. Will she shake my hand? Will she smile? Will she be really nice? She was, and as I faced her with a few other individuals standing beside me, I felt proud and nervous and very excited! What an experience! We were told to call her Your Royal Highness the first time we meet her and then Ma'am (like jam!) any time afterwards. When she spoke to me the 'Her Royal Highness' and 'Ma'am' completely disappeared from my brain and I forgot the names I was supposed to use. Thankfully she didn't seem to mind as I am certain other people will have forgotten this too! Oh well, maybe I will remember if I get this privilege again.

The palace was breath-taking with gorgeous ornaments everywhere. Most of the Royal family had come to this meeting which was fantastic. Camilla was there with the Queen's husband and Princess Anne! I felt overawed because these were faces you are only meant to see on the television set and not in real life. We enjoyed drinks as the Queen made her way around the room speaking to everyone. Yes, the Queen was very nice! On TV she always seemed nice but I had always wondered if it was just a show but this was proof that she was lovely! The Queen walked around the whole team and we introduced ourselves. After she had walked around everyone we were escorted back out of the palace. What a lovely event to meet the Queen and to see her beautiful palace.

I had caught the train to Buckingham Palace with Adrian. Adrian was allowed to walk me to the steps of the palace but had to stop there and was then followed back out of the security barriers by the security guards. Adrian stayed outside the gates until I came out again a couple of hours later. I was with the rest of the Paralympic team and we all felt so special. When I walked out of the palace I looked over to the barriers and saw Adrian who was all smiles and questions and I hugged him telling him it was fantastic. We caught the train back home again each of us with our smiles covering our faces grinning from ear to ear and both of us wondering if we would ever be invited back to the palace again. What an amazing opportunity and an incredible experience!

CHAPTER 59
Rio de Janeiro World Short Course Championships, 2009

Rio de Janiero, the venue for the 2009 World Short Course Championships! The Olympics are a long course meet where we swim in a 50m swimming pool but this event will be held in a 25m ten-lane pool which just means generally faster times due to more turns. I was so very excited about going to Rio. Rio in my mind is just endless beaches like the infamous Copacabana Beach. So stunning. The flight lasted eleven and a half hours and we either slept or watched films the whole flight. The time difference was only going to be four hours so we didn't really expect to be jet lagged but I suppose four hours difference is still quite a lot. Sleeping and resting was therefore compulsory.

It was pretty humid and muggy when we arrived in Rio and the hotel was clean but nothing in comparison to some of the hotels we had stayed in as a team. Nothing had even nearly prepared me for the journeys to the pool or for the storms, never mind the issues with drug testing and getting costumes on! What a turbulent competition!

We had to wake up at ridiculous times to be able to sit on the coach for a full one-hour drive to the pool for every session. Then obviously we had the full one-hour drive after the session to get back to the hotel for lunch. We did two sessions a day which meant we were sat on the bus for four hours solid. The traffic was incredibly slow and we spent a lot of time at a standstill. The food that we were given at the hotel was pretty horrendous (for me anyway!). It was plentiful but we were a little uncertain exactly as to what it was. I am quite a fussy eater so I really struggled to find something I could eat. A number of swimmers complained about the food, that it was over cooked or tasted revolting, but we kept on smiling through all of this adversity! I did find out that the pool we were meant to be racing in had to be closed and we had to use another pool for the competition at the last minute, hence why we had to travel so far.

As part of our travel to the pool we went through favelas which are the slums in Brazil that are most often found in the urban areas. Towards the end of the trip to Brazil, British Swimming took the swimmers to a building in one of the favelas where everyone just danced! The dances were mock fights or defence moves and the dancers were very flexible and strong, each one loving their own dance and their own space! It was incredible to watch and a few people from the team were invited to join the dancers. I watched, amazed how all these people were just enjoying dancing and spending time doing something they found exhilarating! It was a shame when we had to leave and I thought about the lives of these people. They have next-to-nothing but they found so much comfort from this dance that they went to every time they needed it!

Queues everywhere. Queues annoy me quite a lot so this was something I had to try to ignore because there were queues everywhere and for everything. Another thing I hadn't expected apart from the long journey to the pool every day was the weather! I had expected sun, sun and sun but instead we were covered by heavy rain and thunder and lightning storms for many days! The pool was an outdoor pool so the weather made a huge difference. We were not allowed to race when there was lightning and we had to wait for twenty minutes after the lightning before we could touch the water again. For my first race, the 100m Butterfly, the lightning happened just before the race in front of me. I had been all ready for my race with my hat and goggles all in position but instead we had to run and find cover and warmth and then wait for twenty minutes after the storm had stopped before coming out again. My poor body struggled with this new intervention and I didn't really feel ready for my race when it eventually came. My warm-up had seemed such an incredibly long time ago as my race was one of the last of the session. I came third in this race and was expected for my medal presentation but I also had to go to a drug-testing appointment because I had won a medal. I missed this presentation as I did many more during the week just because I was in the drug-testing area either struggling to get my costume off or trying to go to the toilet. Crazy. I would have loved to have gone for my presentations but somebody else had to go to the majority for me.

The weather continued with some very bright sunny days and lots of storms. On one occasion the electricity was knocked out and so we didn't have any electricity for a while. Again we had to sit and wait for the electricity to come back before we could start racing again! One of my races was very interesting because we had to swim with the wind on our side going one way and the wind almost stopping us coming back! An incredible feeling but it did nothing for my coach taking my splits (the times it takes me per length to finish the race): one split was at world record pace and the other was incredibly slow! A large number of swimmers found all of this very hard and they struggled to get fast times. I thought it was incredible that we were meant to race in this kind of weather! In the end, the IPC (International Paralympic Committee) banned swimming outside after this competition saying that all the racing pools need to be under cover from now on.

There was a water lady who was very sweet running around making sure that everybody had enough water! She always had a smile on her face – such a pleasure to meet. One of the problems that all of the swimmers and the British Swimming assistants had during this competition was the costumes. The racing costumes we were using covered the majority of the female swimmer's body (full body suit) leaving just the arms, the feet and the head uncovered. These costumes for speed are meant to be very tight and we therefore chose a size a couple of sizes smaller than our usual one which generally made them near to impossible to get on and off and also very hard to breathe in. In Rio it was very humid because of the changeable weather and with many swimmers all in the same space all trying to get costumes on it was awful. I had to get a few helpers to try to get my costume on, inch by inch or actually millimetre by millimetre. We were all sweating and laughing and pulling and our fingers were cut and bleeding even with the gloves on. We started with the ankles where we often used a plastic bag to help us slide it on more easily. Ankles complete we had just under five foot seven of body left to go! Pull... pull... the calves, knees but then the bum. My bum, thankfully, was quite small so this was never that bad but it was still very hard for us all. The helpers had to bring numerous spare tops so they could have a shower and get changed between sessions. By the time we had got the costume on we had all lost about a stone in body liquid through sweat and grit and determination. The forty minutes of getting the costume on always needed a quick sit down afterwards just to get mentally and physically prepared for the race. We were all so grateful when the full body suits were banned after Rio!

IPC World Championships Results: (25m)

100m Freestyle (S9)	1:01.95	(WR)GOLD
400m Freestyle (S9)	4:39.18	SILVER
100m Backstroke (S9)	1:09.66	SILVER
100m Butterfly (SB9)	1:09.24	BRONZE
100m Individual Medley (SM9)	1:12.61	SILVER
200m Individual Medley (SM9)	2:33.18	GOLD
4x100m Freestyle Relay (34pts)	4:26.20	GOLD
4x100m Medley Relay (34pts)	4:56.23	GOLD

I was quite pleased with these results but don't think I will ever do as many races at one meet again as I was truly exhausted by the end of it!

After the competition we were taken to the giant statue based in Rio which is meant to watch over the whole of Rio. The statue sits on top of Corcovado mountain (which means 'hunchback'), and Cristo Redentor (Christ the Redeemer) gazes out over Rio with a placid expression on his well-crafted face. The mountain rises straight up from the city to 710m and at night the brightly-lit 38m high statue is visible from nearly every part of the city - all 1145 tons of the open-armed redeemer. It was amazing to be a part of such a big feature and we all took loads of photos, amazed at the size of this creature standing in his place looking over the whole of his land and his people! This is now named as the seventh wonder of the world - Sugarloaf Mountain, with its cable car which is used during carnivals. There is also the Maracana Stadium in Rio, which is one of the world's largest football stadiums! We loved the whole day's activities and loved all the photos. Rio is amazing!

Rio de Janeiro will host 2016's Summer Olympics and Paralympic Games which means that for the first time a South American and Portuguese-speaking nation will host the event, although it will be the third time the Olympics are held in a Southern Hemisphere city. In 2014 Rio hosted the 2014 FIFA World Cup so Rio has two years before its huge exposé when it pours its life onto the rest of the world! I expect these Olympic and Paralympic Games and all the celebrations around them to be incredible. It will be a giant party with everybody singing and dancing and colours covering the whole country. Brazil will try to make its mark on the rest of the world the whole way through the Games, congratulating and ensuring happiness through every part of it! It will be fun and everybody will be invited. Smiles are necessary! Dreams are open and free for everybody. Rio de Janiero, the year 2016, the Olympics of a lifetime!

Rio and its World Championships was a very unusual, slightly difficult competition but it taught me loads of valuable lessons and gave me some lovely memories of some incredible events. I now know what to expect in 2016 - I will be ready!

CHAPTER 60

Lost in Transit

When I went to Majorca on a training camp with the Great Britain team, my wheelchair called Fredrick (Rick!) was lost in transit. Where it was lost, I'm not sure; possibly the airport, possibly Cardiff, possibly Majorca. Wherever it was, it was most definitely lost!

Although this was quite an inconvenience, I wasn't overly concerned as my coach, Billy Pye, said he thought that we had full insurance with British Swimming. This would amount to £2,500, and therefore cover the cost of a new wheelchair. Then Colin Bush told me about his friend, Marcus, who wished to start a carbon wheelchair company. Carbon is very lightweight and the wheelchairs would therefore be lighter, faster and easier to manoeuvre. I met Marcus and he talked me into agreeing to him building me a new chair. I would pay him from the insurance money, when it arrived, and in addition to this I would do some promotion work for Marcus, to cover costs.

Little did I know that my problems were just beginning! I sent off the paperwork in order to claim the insurance money, and this paperwork was not received by the insurance company. To make matters worse, I'd mistakenly forgotten to make copies of what I'd sent off.

I could not return the chair to Marcus because he had apparently fitted the chair perfectly in size for me and by now seven months had passed and he had not received a penny. British Swimming were trying their best to get the money for me, and Marcus was stressed as the cost of the wheelchair had already reached £1,600.

This still meant, however, that I was £1,100 out of pocket. Colin Bush said that if I could get someone closer to home to help out, he would give me £500 sponsorship towards the cost of the wheelchair. To top it all off, I had to get brakes fitted to the chair, and this would cost me a further £400-£500.

All in all, this was a very stressful time for me. One thing I did learn from this event was to be selfish. I have to ensure that I take my new wheelchair exactly where I need it so that the airport does not lose it again. I also have to ensure that my name is all over the new chair so that people don't sit in it while I'm trying to get through security. (This happened to me once and it really annoyed me as I thought I'd lost the chair again but someone merely thought it was a great place to sit and rest their legs.)

Thankfully, I've got a new wheelchair now called Rio, but it really was a difficult time for me and for everyone concerned. Extra stress equals extra inflammation on my brain which equals to extra loss of brain cells and inevitably extra loss of my wonderful memories. The MS attacks were expected after this period of stress but in the end I got a wonderful wheelchair thanks to Marcus and British Swimming!

CHAPTER 61

Commonwealth Games, Delhi, 2010

Trials for the Commonwealth Games were complete and the invitation had arrived at my house: I was in the England team on my way to the Commonwealth Games in Delhi, India. To add to this achievement I was the only disabled female who had made the team. How amazing! I felt so proud of this but a little worried that I would feel left out! I was to be a part of the able-bodied England team with just me as a disabled addition and a couple of Paralympic male swimmers who had also made the team. I needn't have worried because my roommate, Stacey Tadd, was so welcoming and so amazing; we had so much fun and really enjoyed each other's company. Billy Pye had to come with me as my coach. Billy is Welsh and he had to be a part of the England team even though he was very Welsh. Billy and I received loads of team kit with England written all over it. I felt especially proud of this. Even though I was disabled I would be in the team with all the able-bodied swimmers. I was almost back where I had left off when the MS attacked. This is almost my able life back on track. I was so excited to be back. England. England kit. Not England-Paralympic-knocked-down-with-MS disabled kit, England able-bodied kit!

The holding camp for Delhi was in Qatar which is in Saudi

Arabia! I was going back to my birth place which I felt so happy about. Would it be like my memories of Jeddah and of all those wonderful times I had there? Would it be roasting hot like in my memories? Roasting hot, yes! Like my memories, kind of! The area and the streets in Qatar seemed the same as Jeddah with the same dust and the same buildings and mosques everywhere, the Arabs walking around with their white cloths which almost look like a uniform to stay cool. The females were all covered in their black abaya, which is a long black robe that covers their body and a hijab which covers their face. I remembered these from Jeddah and they felt very familiar to me.

Our training venue was an incredible facility with under cover football pitches, running tracks and swimming pool after swimming pool! It was an amazing place and I felt so privileged to be able to train there! The hotel where we stayed was absolutely stunning and they had blue crystal seats that I almost didn't want to sit on in case I broke them. I felt so incredibly important and special. I absolutely loved the holding camp and felt very refreshed and ready for my races and my trip to India.

Delhi was so exciting. It is also another venue I can tick off my area list. I have now been to India and have gone back to Saudi Arabia for the holding camp after all this time! Amazing!

Delhi 2010 Commonwealth Games Village
Near Akshardham Temple
Delhi 110092
INDIA

Travelling to the swimming pool from the Commonwealth village was quite an experience as we had armed guards on the bus with us. It was so exciting! We had gunmen everywhere. There were gunmen on the buses in front of us, gunmen on the bus with us and gunmen behind us - incredible. We stayed in the village quite close to the Taj Mahal which is one of the places in the world everyone has to see. I was so impressed by the stunning building. India seems to be one of those places which has a huge rich and poor divide where you can see the amazing, expensive buildings but then also see the naked children by the side of the road. The poverty is a real shame and as ever I wished to help them all.

Something that Delhi is renowned for is Delhi Belly! Delhi Belly is sickness and diarrhoea. We had been given a warning that Delhi Belly was caused by food with sauces so therefore I ate next-to-nothing. I was very worried about this so I stayed very meticulous about anything I ate making sure that nothing had anything resembling a sauce! In the end all I ate was plain pasta and pizza! I lost quite a lot of weight but I don't think it mattered because I didn't get sick. Half the squad, however, did get sick and just listening to conversations was quite revolting with all the good swimmers being knocked down by this bug that we had been pre-warned about. I was so glad I hadn't listened to my hungry belly that was saying 'You will be fine' and instead listened to my brain which said 'Listen to the warnings.'

The Commonwealth site was incredible and something that amazed me was that when there were too many monkeys on the site the wardens had to bring apes onto the site on the end of a leash to scare or get rid of some of the monkeys! This seems crazy but definitely made me feel very special and lucky that I was in India. A once in a lifetime experience I am sure.

HRH Prince Charles came and watched us train in the outdoor pool which was in the village and said how lovely we all were. I felt so proud that a member of the Royal family had come all this way to wish us good luck. The outdoor pool, however, was very dirty with all sorts of creatures floating around dead in the water.

My room was very bare but we were all given a Delhi Commonwealth Games single duvet cover and pillow case which most of us took home to show our parents and keep as good memento. A wonderful souvenir of a wonderful memory. The room, however, was very basic and not quite finished as the showers were without tiles. It was so strange not to have everything that a normal hotel room would have and it made the whole experience seem extra special. Stacey and I laughed and laughed when we noticed the parts of the room that were only a little complete.

All the helpers in Delhi tried their hardest and always were smiling and wanted us to enjoy our stay. Good job guys - Stacey and I loved our stay.

The races that I swam in were very exciting!. As a disabled S9 classification female swimmer I was only allowed to swim three events: 100m Butterfly, 100m Freestyle and 50m Freestyle. There were no other classifications competing there at all for females. The male disabled swimmers were a little more fortunate as they could take three swimmers from three different classifications - S8, S9 and S10 - for different events. I felt very special though being the only disabled girl swimming for England.

I came second in both the 100m Freestyle and the 100m Butterfly races which I was very proud of. Something really weird happened, though, in my third race, the 50m Freestyle. The swimmers had all been called up ready to start the final but somebody did a false start, the gun went so I started and swam on noticing that nobody was swimming the race with me. Looking around on both sides I wondered what on earth had happened. I stopped swimming to see that nobody else had dived in. What? The gun had sounded. I swam over to the wall and climbed out with one of the England team helpers helping me to stand.

'What on earth happened then?' I asked, very annoyed that I would have to re-swim the race.

'Stephanie, you should have finished the race because then the other swimmers would have all been disqualified. You did everything right.' (Surprise, surprise).

In the end I only won a bronze medal for the 50m Freestyle but truthfully I had had to swim further than everybody else. I was awarded a medal and a scarf for winning my two second and one third place medals! I gave one of the scarves to Stacey because she had been such a great roommate and one to my dad for his support and because although he was a very well-travelled person he had always wanted to go to India but had never had the opportunity.

Something that I will remember forever was the naked children on the roads. The children had nothing. I felt so sorry for them and looking up I saw a monkey in the tree. At least the monkey had a home and could catch some food. These children had nothing. Billy Pye did a lovely thing by going into a very dirty hidden slum close to the Commonwealth competition site. After the competition and closing ceremony he gave a lot of his Commonwealth kit and some bottles of water to the families living there. They loved these presents and smiled and waved as Billy left the area. At long last somebody wanted to help them! At long last they were not alone! He was violently sick after his visit with the putrid smell of human faeces that lingered in his mind for days. His thoughts still go back to the awful smell and the lack of anything, absolutely anything. Billy kept telling us about this particular child's smile and I wish I had gone with him. It would have been something I would have treasured forever, giving someone something that will make them happy even if it was only for a few hours.

For the next Commonwealth Games in Glasgow, 2014, S9 females were given 100m Breaststroke as the main race so I didn't compete in this competition. It feels so strange to only be considered as an 'add-on' to the able-bodied Commonwealth Games. Maybe one day this will change!

The Commonwealth Games in Delhi was such an incredible experience for me and I loved everything about them! They were a definite learning curve and a chance to see many things I had only ever dreamed about.

Another amazing experience and an incredible opportunity.

CHAPTER 62

House of Commons (again!) and Mutual Support

I was asked by the MP James Gray, who had taken the post as a patron of Mutual Support (the Armed forces MS support group) after our fight to get Betaferon, to go to the House of Commons again to do a speech in front of a few other MS sufferers and some interested MPs. My dad and Adrian wanted to come with me so we all turned up at the House of Commons!

One of the MPs invited us all into the stunning government building which was very exciting. We were escorted to a room and Adrian and my dad sat at the back of the room with the other MPs; I sat at the side with a big display screen in the centre. James Gray welcomed us all and said a small speech about how he was a part of the MS support group all because he had met and helped me at the beginning of my MS! It was so strange having an MP re-living our original meeting when I was just seventeen and we were fighting for the drug Betaferon. He commented about how he hadn't even heard of MS before but that now was enjoying getting behind all the societies! James then went on to talk briefly about the other MS sufferers, such as Anne Durham, a multiple Paralympic medallist who is amazing on her incredible Welsh horse.

After James had spoken he invited Anne to speak and she laid out a full display of her medals and described other exciting parts of her life. We listened to her story in amazement. When she sat down I felt the butterflies in my stomach - oh no, my turn! I hadn't written a speech like Anne had but I knew my story very well and so the speech came out without me even batting an eyelid. I showed the audience my latest medals from the Commonwealth Games in Delhi (two silvers and a bronze) and they all looked very interested in my story. It is incredible how everyone has to fight for something, however small. The MS stories were very interesting and at the end Adrian and I started talking to a lady from the Mutual Support organisation who represented MS sufferers who had played their part in the three forces - the army, the navy and the air force - all of whom had fought for our country before having to fight a solo war against MS. Adrian and I were invited to give a speech at one of these Mutual Support events in Birmingham and we obviously agreed, we were loving being a part of the Mutual Support group and wanted to help in any way possible.

We arrived at the event and I was dressed up in my GB tracksuit ready for my speech. I stood in front of a large number of MS patients: some members were in a wheelchair, others had sticks and there were a few guide dogs which gave their owners some assistance when requested. After speaking to almost everyone in the group I was awarded an honorary membership of the Mutual Support group which I welcomed with open arms! What a lovely gift for me! They wanted me to join them and offer as much inspiration as I could even though I had never fought for Great Britain. How humbling! I felt very proud and very special.

I have since been to a number of Mutual Support meetings around the country and every time I have felt their support. Maybe by me being there and informing them of my successes and my next competitions, just maybe I am helping someone to keep going when times are hard or when the MS pains are just that little bit too unbearable. The other members of the Mutual Support group offer me inspiration whenever I go to see them because they always have a smile on their face. If they can smile even though they struggle to see, talk, walk or move what gives me the right to feel upset whenever I am down? They keep fighting so therefore it is my role to keep fighting too. The pain in my left arm is kind of just in my mind anyway because, as they say, pain is all in the mind, and whenever my legs cease to move it is just because I have overworked them. Well, this might be so! Good planning is all we need. Stay in charge, stay in control, keep smiling and stay happy and positive! Us against the MS. We will WIN!

CHAPTER 63

My Forever Love

He walked in, straight and tall
His blue eyes drifting the crowd
Seeing me smile he came close
A strength I knew, my forever love

His arms squeezing, soothing warmth into me
My life being pulled up tight and sewn together
His lips pressing love into my heart and veins
My world filling with my forever love

He holds me close pushing the pain away
He covers me from the rain or shame
Pulling me in at night, kissing my brow
A strong endless longing, my forever love

He is there for me always, we're destined for life
A family brought forward, out to the world
A hope, a light that will never simmer
An undying, never ending flame, my forever love.

Stephanie Millward Copyright 2000

CHAPTER 64
Altitude Training, Sierra Nevada, 23rd January 2010 – 13th February 2010

Altitude training for me was a new experience. I am still uncertain whether it was a good, worthwhile trip or if it was just a once in a lifetime adventure. In this chapter I will try to explain my ideas about the altitude experience.

Sierra Nevada, Spain. I would have expected the warm sun on my back as I sunbathed on the beach but when I woke up after a two hour coach drive I realised my preconceptions were very wrong, and I realised I was standing on the top of a mountain surrounded by snow and ski slopes. Wow! Spain has always been a holiday destination for me as I love the sun, the sea and inevitable tan! But the views in Sierra Nevada were incredible and even the clouds formed below the hotel! It was breathtaking! Going into the hotel I realised it wasn't just a hotel but more a sports village. There were gyms, sports halls and a six lane fifty metre pool. It was a wonderful place and we, as part of the British team, had been taken here by British Swimming because of the high altitude.

Altitude effects on the body:

The human body can perform best at sea level, where the atmospheric pressure is 101,325 Pa or 1013.25 millibars (or 1 atm, by definition). The concentration of oxygen (O_2) in sea-level air is 20.9%, so the partial pressure of O_2 (pO_2) is 21.136 kPa. In healthy individuals, this saturates haemoglobin, the oxygen-binding red pigment in red blood cells Atmospheric pressure decreases exponentially with altitude while the O_2 fraction remains constant to about 100 km, so pO_2 decreases exponentially with altitude as well. It is about half of its sea-level value at 5,000 m (16,000 ft), the altitude of the Everest Base Camp, and only a third at 8,848 m (29,029 ft), the summit of Mount Everest. When pO_2 drops, the body responds with altitude acclimatization.

The effects of high altitude on humans are considerable. The percentage saturation of haemoglobin with oxygen determines the content of oxygen in our blood. After the human body reaches around 2,100m (7,000ft) above sea-level, the saturation of oxyhaemoglobin begins to plummet. However, the human body has both short-term and long-term adaptations to altitude that allow it to partially compensate for the lack of oxygen. Athletes use these adaptions to help their performance. There is a limit to the level of adaption; mountaineers refer to the altitudes above 8,000m (26,000ft) as the 'death zone', where no human body can acclimatise.

Extract taken from Wikipedia

I stayed in a room with Ellie Simmonds who is a wonderful roommate. We got on very well and laughed often about the smallest of things! She loves music and we spent a lot of our free time downloading songs and then singing along to them! We also spent a lot of our free time fast asleep. Ellie taught me how to download music and I copied all my favourite songs and thanked her every time with a smile and a big hug. I see Ellie as my little superstar! On the first week I had huge hunger pains in my stomach as dinner was at 20:00 having finished swimming by 18:00. I found this hard to accommodate. On this particular day with the hunger pains I ate the same meal as I would otherwise have done and found the pain in my stomach so bad that I had to go see the nurse with two other swimmers, Ellie and Lauren. The nurse kept poking my stomach and asking if it was sore: surely the answer was obvious. The nurse gave me some tablets saying that I had colic and told me not to drink milk and to have only small meals. Colic, I was certain, was an illness that horses got where they have knots in their stomach! Oh well! How was I supposed to keep training if I was to eat only small meals? Well, this worked out better than anticipated because I increased the amount of bread that I was eating which filled me up more.

To make sure we were all still well we had to have blood tests taken during the training camp. I am fine with blood tests so this didn't bother me at all but there were a few people who were scared stiff. I tried to be really strong for everyone informing them that the body would replace the blood that was being taken from us!

The lack of oxygen in the air because we were at 2340m above sea-level was very strange. Going up steps always left Ellie Simmonds and I in fits of giggles just because you get to the top of the steps then you had to stop and recover from the panting before you move on! We thought it was so funny that our bodies were struggling so much up steps! Our bodies and hearts were working a lot harder to transport the oxygen around the body. The body gets used to the lack of oxygen and we produce more red blood cells which therefore gets more oxygen to cells. This would obviously be a positive thing for athletes!

Comments from my diary

Week One

23/01   Travel to Spain. I was very excited and exhilarated as trips are something special and I love travelling away as part of the GB team. I was looking forward to the new feelings being on an altitude camp and the most noticeable thing for me was that the pain I often feel in my left hand disappeared about half-way up the mountain!

24/01   People kept saying how impossible it was to breathe and although I felt quite heavy the breathing was fine for me. In the pool today the swimming was easy and I enjoyed it very much. The only thing I struggled with was going up the stairs after swimming which seemed to exhaust me very much.

25/01   I felt very strong in both sessions today and the whole camp still had the exciting, fresh feeling with everything feeling good.

26/0   1 Travelled to Granada in the morning which was very exciting. I felt very tired and I realised what they had meant by the inability to breathe because when we went back up the mountain I felt heavy and dark. The pain I have in my hand reappeared in Granada, however, but disappeared again on the way back up the mountain. The gym work I did was very hard and all the work I was doing felt twice as hard as it should have done. I felt exhausted without doing any work. The swim session was very, very, very hard. This meant that all the activities of the day had truly exhausted me. I felt annoyed that I was so tired.

27/01   Feeling tired and sore today and when we were eating dinner I had to go to the nurse for a check up because of excruciating pains in my stomach. This was diagnosed as colic, possibly due to the time period we had to wait after swimming before we were given a meal (at 20.00). I was angry that I had fallen ill so early on the camp and I was very frustrated that the main meals were given to us so late. (Siestas should be banned!)

28/01   Felt very tired today but the training went pretty well.

29/01   I swam quite well today and very much enjoyed the swimming.

30/01   Very, very, very hard session today but I enjoyed it.

This first week was very positive and it was a very motivating and exciting time. The sessions were apparently easy but they seemed to be pretty hard in my eyes!

Week Two

01/02   This was very, very, very, very hard swimming as the sessions seemed to have got a bit harder. The breathing seemed to be difficult and the stairs proved difficult all the time.

02/02   I loved this session! It was very good fun and I really enjoyed it. It was a perfect session to raise motivation and to bring my dreams closer!

03/02   I enjoyed this session very much. This week is very good and all the work, although hard, is feeling worthwhile.

04/02   I was full of a cold today which annoyed me. I hate being ill and little illnesses like a cold frustrate me. I was isolated from Ellie which, although was peaceful, frustrated me. The illness had won and my body had given in to a bug.

05/02   This was a hard day because I felt so ill. I was in a very bad temper and everything annoyed me especially two swimmers who did incredibly easy sessions while everyone else worked their socks off. They were disrupting the whole camp because it felt as though they were skiving and having an easy time, as though they were being given special privileges for whatever reason.

06/02   Tired. I was very tired today and I was getting fed up of the 3x200m step test checks.

07/02   Sunday!! Day off!!

I felt I had a good week but I was annoyed about the cold and the way certain people had an easy ride. I was feeling tired and a little stressed where I felt it was almost time to go home in my opinion and everything seemed so difficult

Week Three

8/02   I pulled something in my arm which annoyed me. I have been hit with everything this camp from colic, to a cold and now I had pulled something. I was very frustrated by this point with little things stressing me out. I kicked excessively because of my pulled muscle which although good for my legs killed me! My step test was delayed.

09/02   I kicked all the session again which I enjoyed.

10/02   I started swimming again today and kept the huge proportion of

kick going strong! I did a 3x200m set which I was quite impressed with.

11/02   It was a nice session today. I am getting back into the swing of things and am feeling less frustrated and angry that everything had gone wrong for me.

12/02   Max Heart Rate set today which was pretty exciting but very hard. It was a nice finish to the camp.

13/02   Fly home today. I put one word in my diary. RELIEF. The trip had been good and hopefully all the training had made us stronger and faster but as John Atkinson says, 'Look after the little things and the bigger things will take care of themselves'. I reckon we should exclude the nuisance individuals, as they did not work hard at all or else were very pessimistic. Get rid of the little issues and the big training sessions will seem that much more appealing. To be back home would be exciting as I would be able to breathe. The pain in my hand didn't return straight away.

14/02   Valentine's Day! No comment!

I know this sounds bad but I was grateful to get home. The camp had been hard work both in and out of the pool and everyone had started annoying me. I feel that the training helped to get me very fit and strong and that is a good thing.

Week Four

15/02   Easy day in the pool. I felt so fast and swimming was very enjoyable and very exciting and again I felt so fast.

16/02   I had a bad day but I swam very well feeling especially fast and light in the pool.

17/02   Swimming was good today. I had a very good set and I still felt very light and high in the water and very fast.

18/02   I had a very hard set today but it was fine because I was swimming so well. It was very enjoyable. The MS pain in my hand still hasn't returned since returning from altitude but I am not complaining!

19/02   I was very tired today but I really enjoyed the session as I still felt fast.

20/02   I was very tired again today and I am feeling strong and fast.

21/02   I stayed in bed all day today. I felt exhausted as though I had eventually run out of power. I hate staying in bed and the fact that I had to, frustrated me immensely.

I loved this feeling as I felt so fast and so light, almost as though I was flying or skimming over the top of the water! This was a wonderful week.

Week Five

22/02   I swam very well today; I had good times and I felt very strong.
23/02   I had a nice session today. I am swimming very well and feeling very fast. Felt the MS pain again in my left wrist. Shame, I was enjoying the break!
24/02   The times just weren't there today but the motivation was and I felt strong, irrelevant of the times.
25/02   I had OK sessions today. I enjoyed the swim as I always do but I am feeling a little heavy.
26/02   Swimming was very good today and I am feeling positive about the competition in Sheffield. I am interested in how fast we can go after the altitude camp.
27/02   I had a good session today where we had to race against time to see how many hundreds we could complete before we didn't make the turn-around time. I did twenty-nine and I was pleased with myself!

The light feeling had left me but I still felt very strong and very good and I felt that the camp had been a success; I was looking forward to racing in Sheffield.

Week Six

01/03   Swam very well today and had not anticipated the speed that I achieved! I was very impressed with myself!
02/03   I swam well today and I really enjoyed the session.
03/03   I swam well in the am but I probably pushed myself too hard and I swam appallingly in the pm session and disappointed myself in my step test.

04/03   I felt awful today and my body was shattered. I just felt drained and exhausted.

05/03   It was the drive to Sheffield and I felt OK, neither positive nor negative about the event in Sheffield.

06/03   I swam appallingly. My MS was fighting with me and I had no speed. I felt embarrassed by my times and I was frustrated as I had expected good times and they just were not there.

A disappointing finish to the camp. I had been so confident that the camp would have allowed me to swim fast in Sheffield. This week after two pain free weeks the pain in my hand had come back. I was amazed that it had stayed away so long!

Positive and negative effects of altitude training

Positive Effects
Enjoyed being on a camp

Enjoyed no distractions

Got rid of MS pain in arm/hand

Enjoyed training hard

Enjoyed trying to swim fast
with no ill effects

Something different from the
norm

Exciting to see the results

The text book proves that altitude
works

Exciting to be part of research

Psychologically felt I was doing
something to make me faster

Negative Effects
Felt awful, shattered, worn out

I felt very tired

Found going up stairs very difficult

Frustrated, aggravated

Overview and additional comments

Camps

I enjoyed the camp and think it was a good training project and it helped the majority of the swimmers on the camp. I feel that the camp got me a lot fitter and stronger but I am not sure it helped my speed in any way. The altitude camp may be a good thing to start the year when the body has just had Christmas, has eaten too much and is feeling lazy and larger than usual. I feel that as a swimmer in Swansea where we are generally very strong with aerobic endurance training, the altitude camp was helpful for us as it pushed us when we were feeling tired and fed up.

I am not sure how often we should have an altitude camp - possibly just once a year as I found it exhausting although I loved the feeling when I got back home; light and fast! The best time to have a camp, I feel, is during the hard or aerobic cycles of the year when the training is hard and essential and the more effective red blood cells would help with making the hard sessions easier. I know that the altitude training is meant to make you faster but the effects were not obvious in my case and so I feel more testing would be useful. The research says that the effects of more effective red blood cells may not be apparent after the first altitude session and so therefore maybe I was naive in expecting the speed. I would like to try the altitude camp at least two more times to see and monitor the effects of more camps. The research proves that the altitude theory should work and hence the camps will be a huge success eventually.

Tents

I would love to try an altitude tent as it would give the positive effects of altitude training without the negative ones. I think that the tent would get rid of my MS pains (proven by the majority of MS sufferers) and it would allow us to train with our home comforts to the standard that we normally hit and without the disturbances of people we don't usually train with. The tent would be very convenient and it would be interesting to see how I would cope with the tent. As the tent is a lot more user-friendly than going on an altitude camp I think it would be beneficial to have a tent for a full month to get used to the effects and then for one week during every one or two months to keep the effects going. I feel that the tent would allow you to do all the hard training without the extreme tiredness. I can only think of positive things for the tents therefore a definite thing for the future.

Conclusion

I feel that the altitude camp was a great success even though I didn't swim as fast three weeks after altitude as I had predicted from the research other people have done on altitude and its effects. I find the research and the idea of altitude training very exciting and I would love to find out more about and be involved more with the research into altitude and the results they have already proven. I think that altitude is definitely a thing to help us get faster in the future and although it is expensive I feel it is a great way to use the money. I feel that altitude can benefit us immensely in the future.

After the camp I was allowed to try an altitude tent which proved to be a wonderful experience for me!

CHAPTER 65

Altitude Tent

When the human body is exposed to hypoxia (oxygen reduced environments), it struggles to produce the required amounts of energy with less available oxygen. This struggle triggers the onset of a range of physiological adaptions geared towards enhancing the efficiency of the body's respiratory, cardiovascular and oxygen utilization systems! For me, the reduction in oxygen, either from going to Spain to the altitude camp or from sleeping inside an altitude tent, reduces the pain in my left hand which makes me, or seems to make me, more positive.

With an altitude tent that you hire you can get all the benefits of hypoxic training at a fraction of the cost of buying your own altitude tent and generator. (It's also cheaper than going down routes outside most sports rules!) Hypoxic units cost a lot to buy but they are proven to enhance athletic performance - hypoxic training will give you extra aerobic power in your sport. With the majority of adaption coming after 6-8 weeks, it makes sense to just rent one for 2 months to prepare for a big race! British disability swimming bought two altitude tents and allowed me to use one in the run up to London and again during London 2012 Paralympic Games! The altitude tent always got rid of the pain I experience in my left hand and arm especially, and after I had been sleeping in the tent I always woke up in a great mood! Adrian tried sleeping in it once. It made him so ill - similar to the symptoms of Man Flu, which are apparently awful. I know of a few people who have Multiple Sclerosis who have either adapted their room to enable them to sleep at altitude or they have bought an altitude tent especially, because it does relieve the pain symptoms.

Altitude training, i.e. hypoxic training which is training with less oxygen and therefore is just like being at altitude, involves exercising in, living in or otherwise breathing oxygen reduced air to improve athletic performance, pre-acclimatisation to altitude and/or physical wellness. Until quite recently when the altitude tents were invented you would have to travel to or live at high altitude to obtain the benefits of this phenomenon. In the mid-90s a company called Hypoxico eliminated this by allowing high altitude training experiences to be set up anywhere. Through the production of hypoxic (oxygen reduced) air, and a tent, it is possible to simulate altitudes of up to 21,000ft/6,400m in your front room or bedroom! As a result, you can have the benefits associated with altitude training while at sea-level in easy places such as your home!

The proven benefits are as follows: Improves speed and endurance, increases strength and power and improves energy levels and overall wellness. Anyone can benefit, but especially athletes and mountaineers!

I found the altitude tent very useful as a psychological advantage as well as a physical one. When British Swimming asked if I wanted to be able to use an altitude tent during the Paralympics in London I thought it would definitely help me. In the end, the Games Makers drove me to a university close to the Olympic Village, where the altitude tent was being stored and I stayed inside the tent for a certain period of time before coming back out and being driven back to the Olympic Village by the Games Makers. I made some wonderful friends both through the Games Makers but also at the university. What a lovely, different experience.

Did it help my racing chances? No idea but it got rid of my pain in my left arm. Did it make me any faster? Probably not but it did what it was there to do and eliminated my pain! Would I use the tent again at a competition? Probably not, because it was just an extra thing to think about but it was a very new and different experience for me.

Altitude tents are amazing.

CHAPTER 66
Naked Photos

I had never thought that anyone would want a picture of me without any clothes on! Clothes are necessary for everything! Why would they want a picture of me wearing absolutely nothing? Well, the national newspaper, the Daily Mail, did want this picture both of me and eleven other athletes! This picture was seen as good promotion for the fast approaching London Olympic and Paralympic Games 2012. I agreed and travelled to Essex.

When I arrived in Essex everything was very professional. We were given a dressing gown to get changed into and were given time slots for our photo shoot. I was very nervous because obviously I had no experience of this ever before. The swimming pool that was used for the underwater shots was the same venue that was used for the incredible film 'Titanic'. I therefore was swimming in the same water as Leonardo DiCaprio!

I got undressed and stood ready behind the closed door until I was called in. The photo shoots were organised so well that I only quickly saw a couple of other athletes either arriving or leaving the venue. It was done so well that you didn't see a whole load of naked people hanging around. Now was my turn. My stomach had huge butterflies as I felt excited and nervous. 'They have seen naked people before, it will be fine,' I kept telling myself.

I walked into the room and saw the pool in front of me with steps leading down. There were three men there in their places. I took off my dressing gown which felt almost unreal. People were going to see me without any clothes on? How can I do this, it is so strange. Truthfully I walk around in a swimming costume for a lot of the day so just minus the costume actually was easy. Everything was done so professionally and it seemed like I was posing with clothes on even though I was naked and underneath the water! The three men were necessary. One had a breathing mask which I could take breaths from when I needed to and the man held it close ready for me. The second man made sure I didn't drown when he tied my ankle to the bottom of the pool to hold me down and the third man took the pictures. All I had to do was pose! All the areas that needed to be covered for the final picture were obstructed by bubbles or my arm if I posed in the correct way. What an incredible experience. The whole process was over in minutes but I enjoyed every second of it. What a fantastic opportunity that I am certain I won't do again.

After the photo shoot we were taken to another room to look at the pictures – how strange! It didn't seem like the photos were of me! My hair was wet (obviously) so I looked different to normal photos, and it was floating up in the air by the water that was surrounding it. The photos were amazing and we chose the perfect one. My hair looked crazy but I enjoyed the end result very much! The final photo can be found on the internet. The picture went down a storm and it was all over the paper and in the lads' magazine 'Nuts!'

This was an experience that always makes me smile when I remember it. It has given me an insight into what a glamour model has to go through for their job! I had a great time and was buzzing when I caught the train home!

CHAPTER 67
Open Meets and Working Abroad

I love the fact that as part of my job I get sent to all sorts of different countries either to compete or to go to a training camp. I feel so lucky.

IPC European Championships, Iceland

Iceland? Land of Ice? Freezing? Iceland is definitely not a place to go if you struggle with the cold! The warm-up pool was outside in minus temperatures and we had to run to get into the pool before we caught frost bite! The racing pool was inside and pretty stunning but if you were swimming backstroke you had to make sure you didn't watch the lines on the ceiling as you would be swimming into the lane ropes all the time. I swam very well at this meet, winning loads and loving the exciting runs to the pool to warm up. We were all given gorgeous coats as part of our team kit to help with the cold, which we wore most of the time! Princess Diana had apparently stayed in the same hotel as the Great Britain team did which I felt was an immense honour. In Iceland I won five golds and many European records.

This was a very exciting event. We were also lucky enough to see the Northern Lights which are an incredible sight! The Northern Lights are the result of collisions between gaseous particles in the earth's atmosphere with charged particles released from the sun's atmosphere. We saw many variations in colour which are due to the type of gas particles that are colliding. The most common aurora colour, a pale yellowish-green, is produced by oxygen molecules which are located about sixty miles above the earth. The bright dancing lights of the aurora are actually collisions between electrically charged particles from the sun that enter the earth's atmosphere. The lights are seen above the magnetic poles of the northern and southern hemispheres. They are known as 'Aurora borealis' in the north and 'Aurora australis' in the south. These were so dramatically beautiful and definitely worth seeing if you get the opportunity. They were amazing!

The Netherlands

The GB team went to the Netherlands on a training camp in 2009 and I really enjoyed the whole experience. The purpose of our trip was to visit two hotels the year before the World Championships, to see which hotel we preferred. Obviously we loved this camp and chose this hotel because it was so luxurious.

Peter van den Hoogenband, who was an incredible swimmer from the Netherlands, has a pool named after him. This pool is in Eindhoven and was the perfect venue for the IPC World Championships in 2010. I felt so important swimming in this stunning pool. I swam well in Eindhoven, winning five silver medals and one bronze. A good medal haul for my World Championships.

There was a lovely barbecue and party after the competition, held on the field by the swimming pool. There was a huge barbecue and a disco so therefore lots of dancing. I had a great time especially when I was dancing with a number of blind people from different countries.

I stayed in a room with Ellie Simmonds, with whom I stayed many times during our careers. I seem to get on very well with Ellie as we seem to suit each other's personalities. Ellie learned from my experience and I found myself re-living age seventeen in a brighter, happier light! Ellie always makes me smile and we have deep and meaningful chats before we wish each other sweet dreams and fall fast asleep.

Majorca and Cyprus training camps

The Great Britain team were invited to warm weather training camps, often visiting venues such as Majorca or Cyprus. On one occasion I was invited to go to Majorca on a training camp. The venue BEST is owned by two past Olympic swimmers who were lovely. The hotel we used was called Blau and was just a short walk from the pool and the adjoining gym. This was perfect for the team who were given specific slots for the gym sessions and then for the pool sessions too. The pool was a 50m pool which is Olympic/Paralympic sized. This long course training is perfect as it is harder work to swim the full 50m without a turn or a break! I loved these warm weather training camps as I loved being away from home where there is nothing to think or worry about. Basically the food is available, the bed is available and all you have to do in return is train hard! The sun is also incredible and I often came back very tanned! These training camps made me feel so important and so special!

IPC World
My current personal bests

Event	Time	Year	Record
Long Course S9 50m Freestyle	29.63	2009	
Long Course S9 100m Freestyle	1:03.18	2009	
Long Course S9 200m Freestyle	2:17.00	2009	ER
Long Course S9 400m Freestyle	4:40.01	2012	ER
Long Course S9 50m Backstroke	33.54	2010	WR
Long Course S9 100m Backstroke	1:10.20	2009	ER
Long Course S9 200m Backstroke	2:34.56	2008	BR
Long Course S9 100m Butterfly	1:10.61	2009	
Long Course SM9 200m Individual Medley	2:36.21	2012	

International competitions I have competed in:

Competition	Event	Year	Time	Medal/Position
Paralympic Games				
	400m Freestyle (S9)	2012	4:40.01	SILVER
	100m Backstroke (S9)		1:11.07	SILVER
	100m Butterfly (S9)		1:12.01	5th
	200m Individual Medley (SM9)		2:36.21	SILVER
	4x100m Freestyle Relay (34pts)		4:24.71	BRONZE
	4x100m Medley Relay 34pts)		4:53.98	SILVER
	50m Freestyle (S9)	2008	30.45	6th
	100m Freestyle (S9)		1:04.52	5th
	100m Backstroke (S9)		1:14.13	4th
	100m Butterfly (S9)		1:15.62	13th
IPC World Championships				
	100m Freestyle (S9)	2013	1:04.00	GOLD
	100m Backstroke (S9)		1:10.56	GOLD
	200m Individual Medley (SM9)		2:40.29	SILVER
	4x100m Freestyle Relay (34pt)		4:27.95	GOLD
	4x100m Medley Relay (34pt)		4:46.21	GOLD
	100m Freestyle (S9)	2010	1:03.85	SILVER
	400m Freestyle (S9)		4:47.04	SILVER
	100m Backstroke (S9)		1:10.31	SILVER
	100m Butterfly (S9)		1:11.07	BRONZE
	4x100m Freestyle Relay (34pts)		4:29.49	SILVER

Competition	Event	Year	Time	Medal/Position
	4x100m Medley Relay (34pts)		5:00.93	SILVER

IPC European Championships

Competition	Event	Year	Time	Medal/Position
	50m Freestyle (S9)	2011	9.95	4th
	100m Freestyle (S9)		1:04.30	SILVER
	400m Freestyle (S9)		4:42.23	GOLD
	100m Backstroke (S9)		1:10.54	GOLD
	100m Butterfly (S9)		1:11.62	SILVER
	4x100m Medley Relay (34pts)		4:52.40	GOLD
	100m Freestyle (S9)	2009	1:03.65	SILVER
	400m Freestyle (S9)		4:43.08	GOLD
	100m Backstroke (S9)		1:10.58	GOLD
	100m Butterfly (S9)		1:10.78	GOLD
	4x100m Freestyle Relay (34pts)		4:33.45	GOLD
	4x100m Medley Relay (34pts)		4:54.47	GOLD

PC World Championships (25m)

Competition	Event	Year	Time	Medal/Position
	100m Freestyle (S9)	2009	1:01.95	GOLD
	400m Freestyle (S9)		4:39.18	SILVER
	100m Backstroke (S9)		1:09.66	SILVER
	100m Butterfly (SB9)		1:09.24	BRONZE
	100m Individual Medley (SM9)		1:12.61	SILVER
	200m Individual Medley (SM9)		2:33.18	GOLD
	4x100m Freestyle (34pts)		Relay 4:26.20	GOLD
	4x100m Medley Relay (34pts)		4:56.23	GOLD

Competition	Event	Year	Time	Medal/Position
Commonwealth Games Delhi	50m Freestyle (S9)	2010	29.69	BRONZE
	100m Freestyle (S9)		1:03.69	SILVER
	100m Butterfly (S9)		1:13.11	SILVER

Domestic events I have competed in:

Competition	Event	Year	Time	Medal/Position
British Championships				
	SM10 200m Individual Medley	2014	2:40.03	5th
	MC 400m Freestyle	2013	4:45.08	4th
	MC 100m Backstroke		1:10.29	GOLD
	MC 50m Freestyle	2012	30.10	BRONZE
	MC 100m Freestyle		1:05.05	6th
	MC 400m Freestyle		4:46.73	6th
	MC 100m Backstroke		1:11.28	BRONZE
	MC 100m Butterfly		1:11.96	SILVER
	MC 50m Freestyle	2011	30.15	BRONZE
	MC 100m Freestyle		1:04.82	4th
	MC 100m Backstroke		1:12.12	GOLD
	MC 100m Butterfly		1:13.62	SILVER
	MC 50m Freestyle	2010	30.87	SILVER
	MC 100m Backstroke		1:10.73	SILVER
	MC 100m Freestyle	2009	1:04.16	BRONZE
	MC 100m Butterfly		1:11.96	SILVER
	MC 50m Freestyle	2008	30:87	6th
	MC 100m Backstroke		1:12.18	BRONZE
	MC 100m Butterfly		1:13.91	BRONZE

Competition	Event	Year	Time	Medal/Position
British Para-Swimming International Meet				
	MC 100m Freestyle	2014	1:04.63	7th
	MC 200m Individual Medley		2:41.11	9th
British International Disability Championships				
	MC 100m Freestyle	2013	1:05.24	BRONZE
	MC 400m Freestyle		4:49.49	7th
	MC 100m Backstroke		1:12.38	7th
	MC 100m Backstroke	2012	1:10.40	4th
	MC 100m Butterfly		1:12.58	4th
	MC 50m Freestyle	2011	30.51	6th
	MC 100m Freestyle		1:05.76	6th
	MC 100m Backstroke		1:11.74	SILVER
	MC 100m Freestyle	2009	1:03.85	SILVER
	MC 100m Butterfly	2009	1:11.47	BRONZE

A new addition to this list is my success at the IPC European Championships. This was held in the wonderful pool in Eindhoven in 2014. My medal winnings are shown below:

400m Freestyle (S9) 4.41.99 Gold!
100m Freestyle (S9) 1.04.06 Gold!
200m Individual Medley 2.38 Silver
100m Backstroke 1.10.9 Gold!
100m Butterfly 1.12 Bronze
4x100m Freestyle Relay Gold!
4x100m Medley Relay Gold!

In 2015 we have the IPC World Championships in Glasgow, then the ultimate Paralympic Games in Rio in 2016. I am so excited about both competitions!

CHAPTER 68

European Trials, Berlin, 2011

This event started with four nights sleeping in the attitude tent in sunny Manchester as a practice for the Paralympics holding camp. This seemed like an added extra to me and I felt we didn't need the trip to Manchester but apparently this trip was good preparation for the London 2012 Paralympics so therefore we went to Manchester as a trial. Fine, I thought, wondering if really this was necessary as I find the extra journey time to Manchester and then to London an extra burden that shatters my body personally. I stayed positive, however, and enjoyed the naivety of the young swimmers who had just joined the team after qualifying for the Berlin European Trials. I loved their excitement and I loved the smile on their faces whenever we were going to do something new! I felt the excitement through them and looked on with the wisdom that comes from experience.

This European Championships would be different than the last Europeans which were in Eindhoven, the Netherlands where I won five golds. This time I would be sleeping in the altitude tent because I had not had a personal best time since the last Europeans. Will the times I swim here be good or would they just be the same? For the previous three weeks I had been preparing for my 100m Backstroke in a different way by wearing my racing suit in the morning and evening sessions on Fridays (the day of my 100m Backstroke in London 2012), swimming my race warm-up, doing a 100m Backstroke stand-up race on my own and monitoring my time for it.

Week 1 am 1:11.2 and pm 1:11.1

Week 2 am 1:10.8 and pm 1:11.1

Week 3 am 1:10.57 and pm 1:10.7

I found this very exciting and felt that when I would swim my 100m Backstroke race I would be ready for it after so many weeks of practice.

I was struggling a bit with the MS as I couldn't really feel my left hand and had a numb sensation all down my left leg. I also felt horrendously tired after my trip to Berlin for the German open meet there. But other than that I was feeling happy and excited and grateful to be me.

The German open meet was good and I won five S9 gold medals and then in the GB relay won two more gold medals: seven gold medals was not bad! I had one world record on the 50m Backstroke. I just wished it was a useful world record and was not brushed under the carpet like dirt. But as a Paralympian 50m Backstroke, Butterfly and Breaststroke are completely ignored and deemed therefore as useless. After this Berlin Open meet we went to the Europeans very excited!

I swam very well at the European Championships, just loving racing and loving winning medals! I also experienced something very frustrating at the European Trials for the 100m Free Relay. I should have been offered a place on this relay team but it was taken away when I mentioned that I felt a bit sick. The food we had been offered was a bit gross so I wasn't surprised that I felt bad! I was very frustrated that I had been chosen for this team but then they dropped me for an illness that was apparently contagious. Rubbish. I felt a little bit sick most probably from the awful food we had been eating and not from this apparently contagious sick bug. The doctor had thought I was fine to swim but the coach took me out. WWWRRRAAAAHH-HH Why do I bother?! I should have remembered my silence lesson that I learned through the MS. If it is not going to kill you keep it to yourself. In Berlin I also had drug tests after drug test after drug tests and it all seemed a little bit over the top. For crying out loud – give me a break. The drug tests were carried out by two people but there was a huge queue of people who needed their tests. We were all stood in the queue desperate for the loo! The selfish few obviously used whatever excuse they could think of and jumped in front. Hopefully everyone learned some lessons from this competition and hopefully these mistakes won't happen again!

A difficult, but truly successful meet for me. Three gold medals and two silvers – not too bad!

CHAPTER 69

Maisie

How can everything be going so well and then one thing changes and everything starts going so wrong? After returning from the Europeans with my three gold medals and two silver ones I felt strong and good. I went back to Chippenham to see my mum and Maisie (my dog) and enjoyed the few days I had their feeling of being on top of the world!

Maisie was my best friend. She loved me which was obvious by the way she followed me everywhere desperate for a hug, a kiss, a walk. She loved sitting on my lap and 'going under the arm' where I picked her up and generally just took her to the car in preparation for a trip somewhere. Maisie seemed to love going anywhere as long as I was there (although she didn't mind going to the beach even without me as company). Her fascination with the beach has always amazed me as she stays away from the sea as she is not interested in getting wet but just loves the run. She runs up the beach then back, then, if you start to run with her, she will charge off loving the whole experience. This is the reason we were going to scatter her ashes on the beaches in Brean. Her death, however, was a living nightmare.

It had started as a good day. Living in Swansea I don't think I will ever expect this. I swam twice, with the second time being quite quick. Maisie had stayed in bed during the morning session but had wanted to come swimming with me in the afternoon so I let her come and she slept in the car with a tub of water and open windows while I swam. Towards the end of my session I started thinking about Maisie and felt a little anxious for her so I sped my session up and got changed very quickly so I could get out and see Maisie as fast as possible.

Looking through the window I was comforted by seeing her still snoozing on the front seat. Hearing me outside she woke up, stretched and then pushed towards the window ready to reach me. I gave her a big kiss and jumped in the car with her ready to drive up the hill back home. Maisie took up her usual seat on my lap and we set off. I had taken my car in for servicing recently but the car had come back worse and it struggled to change gear even though it was an automatic car. As the car went up the hill I noted how slow it was today and decided to take it to the garage the following day.

Maisie and I got home and cooked a spaghetti bolognese. Maisie, as most other dogs do, loves cheese, so I dropped a few bits which she gobbled up in no time. While I ate my dinner Maisie had a large bowlful of mince with grated cheese on top. Normally I wouldn't have given her this as I know it can't be good for her but thankfully I did feed her with this today. Then Fran O'Connor, my house mate came in. As I had rushed my session I had finished before everyone else so she came in later than me. Fran made a fuss of Maisie then asked if I would like to go to the cinema with Ellie Simmonds and herself, I now wish I had said yes but instead I said, 'No thanks. Maisie and I are going for a walk.'

Maisie and I got ready for our walk: lead, coat. Walking up the hill we were very merry and excitable, saying Hi to the children who were playing on the grass. One of the children came over and said, 'You are the swimmer, aren't you?' and I said yes. He invited me to play but I said I needed to walk Maisie. We trotted off up the hill. The walk was nice as we walked along the main road with a number of cars passing us and about ten or fifteen minutes later we walked back down the hill but this time the cheerful children's laughter was gone and it was very almost deadly quiet. Walking further we saw a man and a lady came out of one of the houses and started they calling for someone. I assumed it was one of the children but was later informed they had been calling for 'Chico', their illegal pit bull terrier.

When Maisie and I reached approximately ten metres from my house the nightmare occurred. A large stocky dog jumped on Maisie's back smashing her to the ground screaming, I started screaming too: get attention, stop this nasty revolting dog! Scream! Maisie was crashing around trying to get away and I was bent over punching the dog in the face screaming with all my might. Get off her, get off, get off, wwwrrrraaaahhhh! I smacked it again and again and grabbed its left ear. Yank, pull, get the dog off Maisie, take him away, pull that ear. There was no collar to grab and no lead. Why wouldn't you keep your dog in some control? Why didn't they lock it in its house? Screaming and fighting I didn't notice when Maisie stopped crying but I kept up my scream. The dog tried to bite me twice but Maisie was inside its mouth so instead I got slobber all over my arm. In some ways I wish it had bitten me, then Maisie would have been elsewhere and maybe alive and then I would have something to show for all the pain and terror I was feeling at the time.

Did the lead get in the way? If she didn't have it on would she have been able to get away? Probably not but these thoughts will run through my mind forever now as we will unfortunately never know if there was a way of saving her. Completely ignorant of all the jabs I was making at it the dog trotted off with its kill in its mouth as a cat would with a mouse! Here, owner, a present for you. I was fuming and when it dropped Maisie on the floor still and dead with her eyes wide open and the look of shock and surprise all over her body.

'Maisie, I love you I am so sorry. I shouldn't have taken you for a walk I am to blame. I am sorry.' I was stroking her body so cold and lifeless. I didn't see the blood stains and I didn't see the open wounds I just wanted to stroke some good into her body to bring her back alive and well. She can't die I can bring her back. Looking at her eyes there was only a dead stare and I knew she had already gone but I keep stroking; get her warm, bring her back.

'I think she just shut her eyes and died.' The policeman was trying to make me feel better and it worked a little bit but now I imagine her shutting her eyes hoping for death and I felt the pain she must have been in. I was no help, screaming for someone, anyone to help and my voice and throat struggled for a couple of days later. My neighbour, Caroline Petrinolis, and her daughter, Fran, were wonderful, putting their arms around me and taking me to their home for a cup of tea. The police were called by Caroline and they were also lovely, digging a grave in my garden although I asked them a few times to check that she was actually dead, to make sure we didn't bury her alive. I knew she was dead but just didn't quite believe it. Adrian and then my mum called me trying to understand what and then why it had happened but I couldn't get my words out through all the tears. Caroline was an angel and she explained it to both of them with me quivering and sobbing and unable to understand why it had happened. Adrian, after finding out what had happened, drove at breakneck speed to Swansea to put his arms around me, where they would stay for days to try to control my tears.

We sat in the house for a bit trying to understand what had happened. Why had it happened? Everything was wrong. I had just gone for a walk with my dog and a pit bull had attacked. Pit bulls are a banned breed. Why would it be in Swansea on my road attacking my dog? This was all so unreal. The dog is banned. Adrian started driving back to my mum's house in my car which was desperate for a service. We arrived to see my mum and her partner Nick Woodall at quarter to one in the morning and we all hugged and cried.

'Mum, we have not brought Maisie back with us. She is still in Swansea underneath the ground. I can never bring her home again she has gone now.'

I shut my eyes that night and for many nights later and I kept hearing Maisie screaming for help.

My friend Mark Rose drove to Swansea and later dug Maisie up to bring her home to England where we took her to the vet to be cremated so we could scatter her ashes on the beaches in Brean. I didn't go back to Swansea for a number of weeks. I didn't want to replay the memories that were running round my head. I didn't want to feel useless and helpless again.

Peter, my sports agent at the time, and Andy Milton, my friend, went straight to the press. 'We have a huge story.' The press thought this sounded like a good idea.

We sat and chatted to the RSPCA, the police and to anyone who knew something about dangerous dogs. In the end the police got the dog that killed Maisie and they took the owners to court for having an illegal dog and for its incorrect handling – no lead, no collar. My family put it all over Facebook with gorgeous pictures of Maisie, RIP Maisie, and these made me feel stronger but brought all the tears flooding out again. I had a competition the week after Maisie's death so this was another reason we kept it out of the press, that and the fact that the police needed to be left to do their job - first to capture all the dogs and to arrest the owner.

The competition went well starting with the 400m Freestyle. Ellie Simmonds had already hugged me and told me how much they had all thought about me and how much they missed me. Then Maisie came into the conversation and Ellie changed the subject when she saw the tears come into my eyes. Again when I was standing behind the blocks I thought I was going to do this for Maisie and another tear dropped from my eyes before I brushed them away and started focusing ready for my race. The race was nice with an easy speed and I won the heat with metres to spare. I was in the final but I decided to drop out which would allow Fran who was first reserve another chance to get her qualifying time as I already had made mine. I felt nice for doing this and was rewarded by winning two golds before coming home ready to grieve for Maisie.

The beach we scattered her ashes on was stunning, the perfect place for Maisie. The rain covered the ground and I felt it was just right for her. I scattered Maisie's ashes thinking about all the wonderful things we had done together and I thanked her in my mind for all the support she had been for me whenever I needed her. I told her that she will be able to run on the beach all the time and chase seagulls! Maisie had chased a seagull before and it dropped a chicken sandwich that it had picked up. Maisie loved that chicken sandwich even when my mum chased her to try to clear up the mess. The sandwich must have been twice the size of Maisie's head which made it all look so funny! After scattering all the ashes I turned away and walked up the beach. Maisie had loved this area and as if to prove this theory the rain stopped and the sun came out. A pathetic fallacy. I was sure that was just one of the effects used in the movies but obviously it happens in real life too.

My mum bought Adrian and me a large piece of chocolate cake and a cup of tea and we sat in the café thinking about Maisie and about the rest of my family who had not been around to say good-bye. I felt better after my tears and I felt that the nightmares would stop soon as I gradually came to terms with the loss of Maisie. I did wonder about the dog that had killed Maisie and whether it was right to kill this dog because really it had been the owner's fault for having no control. My mum and Adrian convinced me that if it hadn't been Maisie it would have been one of those children who were playing on the grass. The dog was unsafe. Hopefully the police would do well in the court case and win the right to do whatever they needed to. In the end, and just before the Paralympics, I found out that the owner of the dog had lost the court case and that the dog would be put down. The owner also had to pay for the cost of the court proceedings and give me four hundred pounds as compensation. It was this amount as this is what we had originally paid for Maisie. Four hundred pounds for a life, for all the nightmares I had to endure and four hundred pounds for all the tears I had to cry.

Four hundred pounds because someone didn't put a collar on their dog. I don't expect I will receive this money anyway as there will be an excuse why he can't afford it - I need to feed myself and my family and I need to buy another lowlife dog who can fight and win money and obvious respect for me. I can't waste four hundred pounds on a broken heart.

Adrian and I were walking from my car to the swimming pool for training at Bath University some time later and I heard the sound of a dog running towards us from behind. I grabbed Adrian's arm scared stiff; the memories had been stirred. Adrian hugged me saying it was all ok; the dog was just a labrador coming to say Hello. I burst into tears re-living in my mind the revolting pit bull running away with Maisie - his kill - in his mouth. Two years after Maisie's murder I have a fear of large dogs especially the ones not wearing a lead as it is a painful reminder of that awful day. Please put a lead on your dog even if it is a well-trained lovely labrador who has never done anything bad in its life. It is your dog not mine and loose dogs stir up all of my memories.

I also have a garden which I enjoy working in and when I spotted two dog poos on it I also burst out crying. I am not sure which dog it was that had come into my garden to relieve themselves but again it is your dog mess not mine so put your dog on their lead and keep it off my garden. Thank you. I always wanted to save all the dogs and was going to own a dogs' home later in life so no dog had to be put down and every dog had a home but now I can barely even look at dogs without feeling the terror or my tears. I have lost my love for dogs because of a revolting pit bull and its revolting owner.

I have a large picture of me dressed in a GB tracksuit carrying Maisie which sits at the end of my bed. Every night I look over to her and say 'Goodnight Maisie' believing, or rather hoping, she will be able to hear me. I am sure she would smile back in return then roll over fast asleep. Rest in peace Maisie Molly Summer Love Millward (her show name). Rest in peace!

CHAPTER 70

South Africa – Training Camp

One of the highlights of my swimming career as a Paralympian was to fly out with the British team, to train in South Africa prior to the London 2012 Olympics. South Africa is known by its people as the 'Rainbow Nation', due to the many different cultures and language groups living there. To me, the name 'Rainbow Nation' was a wonderful description of South Africa itself, not just the people living there who were amazing but of the whole area that we stayed in. My memories are of bright rainbow colours - the dazzling, golden sun, the cloudless, sapphire blue skies, the green leaves of the palm trees that waved their welcome to us, in the slight breeze. I loved every minute of it!

It was a long flight there - over eleven hours - but for me the trip to another country has always been an enjoyable experience as I look forward to every new adventure and I love the plane journey! When we stepped out of the air-conditioned airport, the heat hit me and it reminded me of stepping out of the airports in Jeddah when my whole family commented on the blast of hot air hitting us. What a lovely reminder. We were visiting during the height of South Africa's summer and our base was located on the hot and humid east coast, near the port city of Durban, in a plush suburb called La Lucia.

We stayed at the Beverly Hills Hotel in La Lucia as this was within easy reach of the Crawford Olympic-sized swimming pool as well as the Northwood gymnasium which we used as part of our training camp. Both venues were perfect for the team's training. We were able to dedicate our time solely to focusing on our swimming in preparation for the 2012 Olympics. This is the whole point of training camps; they help athletes before a competition devote themselves entirely to their sport, without the distractions of normal life.

Our meals were varied and healthy. We had to eat lots of protein and carbohydrates generally before each swim session, and then throughout the day, for energy. We had to also eat protein after each training session in order for our muscles to have the nutrients to enable them to break down and then rebuild again. This type of eating is important to what is called 'Adaption Training', and this type of training is often used before a competition by athletes to induce greater muscle strength. The mitochondria within the muscle are broken down as the athlete overworks themselves - in my case through intensive weight training and swim sessions. The muscle then rebuilds itself much stronger than before.

It was lovely, however, to enjoy the sights and sounds of another country while we trained and during our breaks. The people were outgoing and welcoming, and one of the highlights of the trip was when the staff at the hotel put on a Zulu dance for the team. (The Zulu people populate the East Coast of South Africa and are descendants of the great warrior king, Shaka Zulu.) For the dance they wore brightly coloured beads that glistened and clicked against their chocolate-coloured skin, as well as grass skirts that rustled rhythmically to the beat of the cowhide drums. They sang as they danced, their voices rising and falling in a powerful yet harmonious sound. The GB team absolutely loved it!

Besides the sounds of the Zulu dancers, I cannot forget the sounds of the millions of little insects which struck up their orchestra every humid, black evening as the sun dipped behind the sea. These tiny creatures seemed to be everywhere; see - through lizards pattering across the walls, moths dancing around the lights of the hotel, and thousands upon thousands of invisible crickets under the star-studded sky. It really was a tropical paradise and I loved closing my eyes and just listening to their music!!

Unfortunately, we weren't able to swim in the warm waters of the Indian Ocean (the sea that was very close to the hotel), as due to the presence of bull sharks it was dangerous to venture into the sea! There was, however, a pool at the hotel. A large group of birds called Sacred Ibis, (or 'Har Dee Dah' by the locals due to the sound they made), seemed to have adopted this pool as their watering hole. They would keep the staff at the hotel very busy cleaning up after bird poo in the pool!

I also encountered monkeys when I was in South Africa, and these furry grey creatures would scamper across the ground and up into the trees, in large groups. The baby monkeys would hold tight to their mothers' stomachs, whenever a troupe of monkeys was on the march.

My two week training camp in South Africa was a memorable experience and I felt blessed that I could see and enjoy so many sights and sounds. MS might try to limit me, but this training camp was an incredible oasis of refreshment in the desert of disability.

CHAPTER 71

Pre-Paralympics, 2011-12

There is just over a year to go and I am very worried. What will happen if I am not good enough and I come back from London with nothing? What will happen if I get disqualified in my backstroke? Wow, there are a lot of fears but I needed to stay positive. I occasionally see a young lady who is pregnant in the Springfield Swimming pool in Corsham who is expecting her baby on my birthday. I find this very positive. I feel I have to stay positive for her and for the baby as it will share my birthday so we are therefore somehow bonded! The mother has always been very strong for me so I will hopefully swim well for them too. I still have a few things to do this year -European Championships in Berlin and a couple of smaller competitions - so hopefully I will swim well and these will give me the confidence to swim well in London in 2012!

One of the worst symptoms I have with MS is toilet issues/ control - every day is a worry. I make sure I go to the toilet before leaving the house and make sure that I know where the next toilet break will be. This 'issue' had been a problem for all these years since it first started with the onset of MS in 1999. On one of our yearly review trips to Manchester, which is now the headquarters for the Great Britain Paralympic team, all of the Paralympians had to go to four meetings. One of the meetings was a review with the National Performance director and the head coach as well as your own coach. This was always a bit scary because it was like parents' evenings at school where you are not sure what they are going to say about you.

Another meeting was with the team doctor who took our blood to send for a full blood count to check our ferritin, iron and vitamin D levels. We also have meetings with the team physiotherapist to make sure we are happy with our routines and with our S&C workouts. Our last meeting was with a nutritionist who took our weight and then gave us a skin fold test to measure the amount of excess fat you carry on top of your muscles.

At one of my physio meetings I burst out crying when I was telling the physio how much trouble I was having controlling my toilet facilities. When I needed to go I would run desperately to the toilet knowing what would happen if I didn't get there on time. Paul, the physiotherapist at that time, had seen me mention this before and the tears were the wakeup call that something was really wrong. Paul spoke to the National Performance director who agreed that British Swimming could pay for me to see a gynaecologist to see if they could help. I went to this meeting and got checked over with the gynaecologist who informed me that I didn't need to do anymore lower bridge exercises because I was as strong as an ox - cheeky, I thought! He then fixed me with cables which recorded the movement of everything to see if I emptied my bladder fully. The test showed on a computer that my bladder and bowel were having spasms every few seconds and these spasms were what was making me think I needed to go to the toilet again and again. This was the best news he could have given me! I can control or combat spasms!

After this meeting I made a note of how much I was drinking and every time I had a spasm I sat down, relaxed and told myself this is just a spasm and I don't need the toilet. When I thought that a spasm was a correct time to need the toilet I went calmly. I had to monitor how much was in my bladder and I had to physically think about going to the toilet and then relaxing my spasms. Thirteen years of toilet issues finally all calmed down and I can safely say now that I don't have any issues with bladder or bowel control! Again, I used the power of my mind and some monitoring of my body!

One thing that most coaches do for their athletes is to write a program where they do all the hard work and hard training but then taper just before a competition. A taper refers to the practice of reducing exercise in the days before an important competition. Tapering is customary in many endurance sports, such as the marathon, athletics and swimming. For many athletes, a significant period of tapering is essential for their optimal performance. The tapering period frequently lasts as long as a week but can vary according to the sport and on the athlete. Generally, people should have just two tapers a year so these tapers must be thought about and organised perfectly. For London 2012 I had to taper once before the Paralympic Trials and once before the Paralympic Games to optimise my times once to qualify for London and then to swim well in London.

Starting the taper on the week beginning 30.01.2012, I started increasing speed but decreasing the distance covered per week starting from approximately 50,000m per week and reducing this down to 35,000m. Recovery is very important because if you recover faster you will be ready for the next training session or race. I normally swim five individual races per meet which means five heats and generally five finals! I need to make sure my recovery is perfect so I am ready for each race. I also have to make sure I recover enough to help my MS which will definitely tell me when it is too tired so I monitor everything I eat and drink to make sure I don't get too exhausted.

Endurance exercise and high intensity training places a huge physiological stress on the body, which causes the breakdown of muscle proteins and reduced post exercise glycogen (carbohydrate) levels. Recovery after exercise is essential to stimulate protein synthesis and repair damaged muscle. Using a recovery product helps replace energy and electrolyte stores used up and helps muscles adapt to training and enhance future performance. I normally use milk as my recovery drink and because I don't like the taste of milk I add the 'Nesquik' strawberry ingredient to produce a lovely strawberry milkshake!

Your recovery should start within the thirty minutes after exercise because this is when the body is particularly receptive to protein, carbohydrate and fluid intake. As consuming food at this time isn't always practical this milkshake is perfect to help me optimise recovery. One of the team GBR staff members often takes a drop of blood from our ear to measure our lactate levels, which tells us if we have swum down/recovered enough after a race. A lactic acid test is a blood test that measures the level of lactic acid made in the body. Most of it is made by muscle tissue and red blood cells. When the oxygen level in the body is normal, carbohydrate breaks down into water and carbon dioxide. When the oxygen level is low, carbohydrate breaks down for energy and makes lactic acid.

Lactic acid levels get higher during strenuous exercise and this lowers the flow of blood and oxygen throughout the body which is why we get this measured. My scores are normally just over ten after a race but often drop to the optimal under two quite quickly. As a swimmer I always swim down, which means do a number of lengths which includes some short sharp bursts of speed to move the lactate around the blood and some slower easy swimming. My usual swim-down would be approximately 1200m.

Another thing I like to do, although it can prove to be very expensive, is to go and speak to a psychologist. Psychologists are easy to talk to and they make you feel more confident about your race and about how you are going to prepare for the race. I find psychologists so important as part of my races and before London I had to make sure I was ready for everything!

By the time the London 2012 Paralympics Games came I was definitely ready for anything but I didn't realise quite how supportive Great Britain were going to be for us! The crowd, the papers, the radio, my family, all the feelings around the Paralympics were incredible.

Thank you for all your support! I couldn't have asked for anything more!

CHAPTER 72
Coca-Cola

When I saw the advert on the British Swimming website – work experience with Coca-Cola - I didn't really think anything of it because I wasn't going to get a job working for someone quite as incredible as Coca-Cola, was I? I sent my CV anyway and couldn't quite understand it when I received an interview in Loughborough. Adrian and I thought it would just be a fun trip up to Loughborough and went up there all smiles!

The interview was quite exciting because although I did have one interview where a couple of people asked me questions I also had a team work meeting where a group of the interviewees had a task for which we needed to work as part of the team to be able to do it. I found this very interesting as the louder individuals always show their face first giving their opinions. I held back watching until I was certain how to do it then gave my ideas!

At the interview I met Daryl Jelinek for the first time! Daryl was in charge of the Olympic section of Coca-Cola organising all the drinks both for the summer and the winter Olympic Games and eventually Paralympic Games. Daryl is incredible and I will tell you all about him soon! In the end Coca-Cola offered to me many things including work experience, hope, support and they offered me a place on their Academy of Excellence which made me feel so special. As part of the Academy of Excellence I worked with Coca-Cola for two one-week sessions every year for two years running up until London 2012 Paralympics and have therefore worked in different parts of the business and now know how they work. Coca-Cola is a huge business with almost every person in the world knowing what Coke is! What an incredible company!

They apparently picked me and another girl out of all the twenty people who went to the interview because of our personality and drive to do well. I fitted their criteria perfectly and apparently I did exceptionally well at the interview. During the four days that I worked in their offices in Hammersmith, London, I was told that I worked extremely hard! There is a definite link between the elite athlete and the top performers in the business environment and Coca-Cola wanted to join those two types of people together. It was also an inspiration for the company's employees to meet the emerging Olympians. These athletes were the best of the best. Could the sports people give their drive and determination to the employees of Coca-Cola? The answer was yes! Coca-Cola's employees found it very exciting that they were meeting and chatting to and in some cases working with the Olympic athletes for London 2012; the same people they will be cheering on their television sets!! For me it was a similar buzz working for this inspirational company.

Adrian stayed in the hotel all week with me while I worked in London and I came back every evening telling him what I had done and I was so excited about going to work the next day. My work ethic and enthusiasm seemed to promote hope and inspiration into the team and Daryl heard all these positive comments about me and had to come down to see me in action! Daryl was very impressed and we have been good friends ever since! On another occasion Daryl told me all about his children, Joe and Amy, and about how much Amy especially would love to meet me. In the end we went for a Chinese meal and became friends as we all got on so well. Amy is my 'star supporter' (her words) and an incredible friend. We have been all swimming together; Joe was very good and Amy loved me throwing her around in the pool, and we have been for many meals. Daryl also asked me to do a speech for Amy's school as it was an end-of-term presentation evening. I obviously said 'Yes'. Daryl asked me if I would like some help to write the speech and I said 'Yes, please!' so we sat down and Daryl jotted some notes down on the back of an envelope. I still look at these notes and Daryl's tips as they were perfect! The speech in front of the school was very good and I was quite pleased with everything I had said. I was later invited to another school in London to do another speech which also went down well! Thank you, Daryl, for your lovely recommendations and for your excellent tips. I feel so pleased to have met all of the incredible Jelinek family.

27th September 2011 - Inspiring personal best
This project was one of the first that I did for Coca-Cola. I was asked to produce a presentation and then do a speech for a few important members of the Coca-Cola Olympics Team! This was quite hard because Coca-Cola seemed to have everything already. What could I do to make it any better? Something for disabled people like me would be one idea. I knew that Coca-Cola was already a huge sponsor for the Olympics: why couldn't they be a huge sponsor for the Paralympics too? I set off finding out loads of information about important disabled sports people and the lives of disabled people. I found out about the good and bad parts of being disabled in any sports place and I looked at the importance of hand rails on steps to help people down the steps. When my speech came I felt a little nervous but I knew my speech was strong and when I started off by reading a lovely poem which had been written by a girl with cerebral palsy, about her life and her love of sports. I could tell people were interested in what I was saying! I finished the speech and the whole group clapped for me! This was not expected! 'Well done, Stephanie. That was a very good speech!' Perfect!

The team informed me that they had agreed to fund the Paralympics too but were going to wait for a little while before telling everyone. I felt so special that I had been told this important news before the rest of the world found out!

October 2011 - Judging Olympic Torch relay

I had worked my way all around Coca-Cola's business working in different areas, such I standing on the side of the street handing out drinks to people as they rushed to work and sitting in meetings being involved in Skype conversations. I loved working with Coca-Cola. A short time before one of my trips to London to work with Coca-Cola I was sent an email. This email was such an incredible email. Basically, the email asked me to be a part of the judging panel for the Olympic Torch relay! WOW! What an incredible opportunity. When I arrived at Hammersmith to start judging I smiled and smiled and smiled. This was amazing! In one room there were loads of past Olympic torches all on display. Adrian and I went into the room and couldn't believe our eyes. We could touch them and play with them!

'Look at these torches!' Adrian said absolutely amazed by them.

Each one was very individual and I felt so honoured to be stood in that room with all those incredible torches!

The next part was my bit of work where I sat at a table with a computer. The computer showed different people's application forms to carry the Olympic Torch. This was a blind interview really so we didn't know anything about the person making the application whether they were male or female or British or from another country. It was totally blind for fairness of the selection. I had to read their application and give them a score on different aspects of the criteria. Some of the stories were very heart-warming and I scored them very highly and others seemed like they just filled out the form just in case they could be chosen even though they didn't necessarily deserve to be chosen in relation to some other stories. These I scored less well. After I had done all my grading I left the room.

'Adrian some people are incredible you should hear what they have done!' I was overwhelmed by some of the stories!

Another email was sent to me later in the year saying that I had been chosen to carry the Olympic Torch on the Relay and it asked where I would like to carry it. I said thank you very much and Bath but unfortunately the date that the torch was coming through Bath I was on a training camp! In the end Adrian and I and my mum and

Nick Woodall went to Liverpool to watch me carry the torch! What an amazing experience; I will share it with you in chapter 74.

8th December 2011 - Christmas party at the Royal Opera House, Covent Garden

When I received an invitation for me and one other person (Adrian) to attend the Royal Opera House for Coca-Cola's Christmas party I was over the moon! I found a perfect outfit and Adrian and I turned up with smiles on our faces. The three course meal we were served was fantastic and all the excitement was incredible. Half-way through the meal we had a surprise rendition of the musical performed by the Royal Opera House's Orchestra and their vocalists. It was absolutely amazing! Adrian and I had an incredible night listening to somebody playing a harp for us too and then we did a lot of chatting. People were starting to get excited about the London 2012 Olympics which were just round the corner. Thank you again, Coca-Cola, for a wonderful experience!

1st June 2012, Westfield - Dizzee Rascal

When I was asked to go to a shopping centre, Westfield, which was built right next to the Olympic Village I jumped at the chance! Dizzee Rascal, a rapper that loads of people know was going to be there with me, but I had to keep this a secret because the shopping centre could only hold three thousand people and if word got out that Dizzee was going to perform the place would be mayhem! The press seemed to know that something big was going to happen because they kept on asking us who was turning up. The crowd started increasing around the stage that was made up in the centre of the shopping centre! When Dizzee arrived it was time for our appearance! About seven of us athletes walked on to the stage and the compare introduced us and asked us questions about our sport and our ambitions. The thousand-strong crowd cheered every time a new athlete was introduced; they were so good as they really got into the atmosphere! Us athletes were almost the introduction for Dizzee himself who came out all excited! He was jumping around trying to get everyone to sing with him and somebody grabbed his t-shirt and started pulling so everyone else started pulling too. Dizzee loved it!

'BONKERS!!!'

This was another great experience and Adrian and I loved it!

On one of my weeks staying in London I met the marketing team who were full of new ideas to promote Coca-Cola. During this week I was approached by Olivia who was a lovely person. Olivia told me that she was the link with Coca-Cola's charity StreetGames which is a sports charity that brings sport to the doorstep of young people in disadvantaged communities across the UK. Olivia told me that if I wanted to organise a StreetGames event Coca-Cola could fund it for me if they thought it was a good project. A few other sports people had already done this and had chosen one child who won a prize to teach them how to do a specific sport and there was a judo guy who worked with a small group of children to teach them how to do judo.

What could I do? This was such a lovely idea! I would be helping lots of under-privileged children and they would have a great time! I needed to organise something - swimming? As soon as I had something planned I would be able to apply for a bursary so everything needed to be done perfectly. I needed a venue, I needed to produce some paperwork to tell people what I was doing. I needed links to the local paper and I needed to contact the local council because then I could use their help with assistants on the day! This was so exciting! This was a perfect opportunity for me to help more people! I started to write down my notes and ideas

It's a knock out? *Might be too much for the children.*

Swimming Competition? *What would happen if they can't swim?*

Mini Olympics? *There might have been too many sports for one day which is why the Olympics cover such a long period of time!*

Adrian said maybe try a triathlon but this seemed a bit too big for a StreetGames festival. All of these ideas were flying through my head but in the end the most perfect idea stayed. The festival publicity was put onto a flyer. It was amazing.

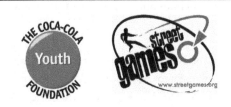

STREETGAMES AND STEPHANIE MILLWARD – AMBASSADOR BURSARY PARTNERSHIP

StreetGames are delighted to confirm that Stephanie Millward has accepted our invitation to become one of our sporting ambassadors. In conjunction with Coca-Cola GB, we are also delighted to announce that Stephanie has been awarded a StreetGames Ambassador Bursary, funded by the Coca-Cola Youth Foundation, to be used to support her local StreetGames project.

We appreciate that Stephanie already has a number of commitments and, that she needs to concentrate on and prepare for the 2012 Games. We are most grateful of Clare's support of StreetGames, do not seek to impinge upon her professional endeavors and are more than happy to work around any existing obligations

StreetGames envisages the following partnership work

To be able to announce on StreetGames and/or Coca-Cola's website Stephanie Millward as one of our sporting ambassadors and her support of *Plash 'n' Sprint* StreetGames project which will receive the bursary.

Stephanie to provide a quote and be available for a short visit to the ambassador's local project (or the location of the initiative they are supporting through the bursary if this is different to the project location) at or near the time of the announcement. We would hope to generate media coverage for this in the form of a one-to-one interview with a national newspaper, national TV station and/or local media. We will also include a photo and/or short online video on StreetGames and Coca-Cola GB's website and/or staff intranet.

Stephanie to answer four brief questions as part of the Bursary Follow-up Report (which is to be completed by the project manager of the local StreetGames project that the bursary has been awarded to) to maximise the benefit of the bursary allocation to other StreetGames projects in the future.

Attendance at a StreetGames Mass Participation or Neighbourhood Festival in 2012 (UK travel costs reimbursed).

To follow Stephanie through StreetGames' social media network – Twitter and Facebook – so that the young people in Street-Games projects can follow his/her career and journey towards London 2012 and send their own messages of support.

Stephanie to follow StreetGames' social media and contribute where appropriate.

To be able to give semi-regular updates for StreetGames' website: www.streetgames.org (ideally monthly but at least every 3 months) on progress throughout 2012. This could be in the form of updates provided by the ambassador or on ambassadors' behalf by their coach or governing body and could include written or video updates, or an informal conversation with us over the phone, whichever the ambassador prefers.

The ambassador to provide us with a typical day's training schedule/work commitments. We feel this has a great relevance to all of the young people in our projects.

Benefits for StreetGames bursary ambassadors

Association with award winning national charity and its partners.

Media opportunities at Street Games events and ambassador sign up announcement to help build ambassador's profile.

Regional/National networking opportunities with StreetGames network, partners and stakeholders.

Access to funding to develop local sporting opportunities in disadvantaged communities close to the ambassadors home or training venue.

Personal development opportunities through the StreetGames Training Academy.

Opportunity for ambassador to attend a media training session in conjunction with Coca-Cola.

Coca-Cola's London 2012 Ambassador gift pack (includes Adidas London 2012 tracksuit top and bottoms, Powerade t-shirt and water bottle).

UK travel costs reimbursed for attendance at Mass Participation Festival.

Adam Smith

I had planned my event, spoken with all the relevant people and had been awarded the money to enable myself and Gareth Govier, a friend from Swansea who worked for the council, to organise this Street Games event at the Wales National Pool in Swansea.

My plan was to choose ten children who were complete non-swimmers and then to teach them how to swim in ten one-hour swimming sessions once a week for ten weeks before I held a StreetGames festival where the children would swim and the non-swimmers would be able to swim with the other children and do all the other sports! It also allowed me the funding to employ a couple of coaches to help me teach the ten non-swimmers with learning difficulties how to swim! It was amazing - thank you Coca-Cola!

The StreetGames festival was organised for the 7th July so ten weeks before the 7th July I went to the pool to meet the ten non-swimmers who we were going to teach to swim. It was such an amazing experience. We went to the smaller 25m pool where we spoke to each of the swimmers about swimming and then we got them in! A couple of the children were scared of water so we worked slowly with them! I went to most of the sessions but I had a training camp and therefore missed two of their sessions but the other coaches were brilliant. By the time the ten weeks were up all of the children could swim well and I was so proud of each and every one of them. The StreetGames event came and there was publicity everywhere with lots of posters up on the walls. I was so excited. We had named the event Splash 'n' Sprint because we were doing other StreetGames activities such as running and ball Games outside on Swansea University's athletic fields as well as swimming!

'Splash 'n' Sprint'
7th July 2012 at the Wales National Pool! Doors opened at 9am and many children signed in and received their StreetGames coloured t-shirt depending on which team they were put in. Unfortunately StreetGames were not able to book a coach to bring the children to the pool so only fifty children were able to get themselves to the pool for this event but that was quite enough! The ten children we had

taught to swim were buzzing and I couldn't wait to see them swim and show everyone else what they had learned! I loved every minute of the day and it was such a shame when it was over. I said goodbye and good luck to each of the ten children we had taught to swim and I asked them to believe in themselves. Anything is possible! A few weeks later I heard that four of the swimmers had started swimming training with one of the local swimming clubs and that another four were having private lessons to get better before they joined a club. I was so incredibly proud of them and so impressed with the success of the whole event.

Thank you Coca-Cola and thank you Street Games and thank you Swansea Council for your help!

CHAPTER 73
Coca-Cola's Academy of Excellence

When I first arrived at the Coca-Cola offices in Hammersmith, the first thing I had to do was to answer a few questions so that they Co-ca-Cola knew who I was! Here is the questionnaire!

Stephanie Millward you were a successful able-bodied swimmer before being diagnosed with MS when you were 17. Your recent achievements have been extremely inspirational. Can you tell us a bit about how you coped with this diagnosis? What effect did it have on you both as an athlete and as a person? It devastated me. I was told that all my dreams were over and that my life was going to go from being a very successful swimmer to being a useless lump of meat in a wheelchair. I could not think of anything worse and I became very depressed by the news. As an athlete I had to stop swimming as I no longer was able to see so therefore could not drive to the pool or walk and therefore could not walk to the pool. My mum took me to the pool once and she was so upset about seeing me struggling to walk that she never took me again after and has only just started watching me racing.

What motivates you? As an able swimmer my motivation came from myself and from other members of my family. We all swam and therefore were our own little team! When I became disabled and lost everything I had initially took for granted my sole support originally was my little Yorkshire terrier, Spring, who would listen to my every word. After a few months my mum became a support as well although it was more her picking up the pieces whenever anything went wrong. I met Adrian McHugh in 2005 and he was the one who got me back into swimming professionally. He kept being positive about how I could still swim as a Paralympic swimmer and that I could train for London so this is what we did. Stardom has never been important for me but I would like to be recognised as a good swimmer

What is your training schedule like at the moment? 9 two-hour sessions in the pool a week plus at least two 1.5 hour gym sessions.

What has your experience of the Coca-Cola Academy of Excellence been like so far? Coca-Cola has been wonderful for me. They have offered me tremendous amounts of support financially and as a person. I am now stronger and more confident then when I first started with Coke and I feel very important being a part of the Academy of Excellence.

How do you feel about being named as one of Coca-Cola's Olympic torchbearers? Delighted! Only 8,000 people in the world have been given places on the torch bearers' route and I am one of those lucky ones! I am so excited about carrying the torch and I can't wait to see the crowds.

What events have you got coming up between now and the Paralympics? I have a two week training camp in Majorca which will be fun but very hard. I am also trying to organise a StreetGames event which should be a bit of fun for the children and for me! I have one competition in Germany in May and then I have London Paralympics! How exciting!

What are your hopes for the London 2012 Paralympic Games?
I have qualified for six individual events and then will probably be asked to swim in two relays as well so that is eight events in ten days. I feel this may be one too many so I will have to discuss with my Coach which seven events I intend to swim! I hope the London Paralympics will offer inspiration to the whole nation and that we all rise and aspire to be athletes and that we all come out after the Paralympics stronger and more determined within ourselves!

I must have pre-seen the effect the 2012 Paralympic Games would have on the whole nation because this is exactly what happened! The whole country supported the Olympic and then the Paralympic teams with all their might yelling and screaming for everyone wearing the GB kit.

Go Great Britain, go!

CHAPTER 74

Carrying the Olympic Torch!

I am not sure what everybody dreams about but carrying the Olympic Torch was miles above any of my dreams. To pick the torch up and inspect the gold rings, all 8,000 of them, shining brightly, each one an indicator of one of the lucky 8,000 people carrying the torch as it makes its way from Athens to Stratford, London ready for the London Olympics 2012 – incredible!

I was on the bus in Huyton, Liverpool excited about my turn carrying the Olympic Torch. All the other runners on the bus had been chatting about why they had been chosen. All the stories were incredible and I felt inspired by every one of them and there were even a few who I remembered as I had chosen them to carry the torch. I didn't remember their names and I hadn't seen their faces but I definitely remembered their stories. Being in the judging panel for Coca-Cola will be something I will treasure forever. When each stood to start their run I felt so proud that I had heard all about them and I knew why they were here carrying their torch!

The man wearing the number 110 had gone out into a crowd of cheers and when he left with the huge smile on his face I started feeling the nervous excitement inside my stomach!

'111 Stephanie Millward. I heard my call and as I stood the cheer from inside the bus was immense!

'Good luck Stephanie and enjoy every second,' I heard someone call after me!

Smiling, I stepped off the bus and was welcomed by a huge crowd who swarmed around me as I moved away from the bus. Everyone was cheering and everyone was smiling. I was carrying my un-lit torch ad I felt so important and so special!

'Can we have a picture?'

'Smile!'

'Stephanie!'

Everyone was calling out to me wanting to get a finger onto the torch, all wanting to be a part of this 2012 Olympic Games.

'Stephanie, can we interview you, please?'

I had requests everywhere and many photos were taken and I tried to let everyone touch the torch! I felt so important and so special and I was overwhelmed that I had been given this wonderful opportunity! I had been chosen to be a part of Coca Colas Academy of Excellence a couple of years ago after a successful interview in Loughborough. Being a part of this Academy of Excellence meant that I was invited to work at the Coca-Cola offices in Hammersmith for two one week periods every year! I loved all my experiences with Coke and when I was asked to be a part of the team who judged contestants for the Olympic Torch relay I was dumbstruck!! Wow! This judging episode happened in the Hammersmith offices where all the past Olympic torches were placed on display in their year order. This was stunning and Adrian and I spent a long time inspecting each one feeling very special!!

'Stephanie, can you stand next to my daughter for a picture?'

'Stephanie, we have to start moving 110 will be here soon'

'Stephanie, smile!!'

The police officer tried to calm the crowd, asking for some kind of control.

'Everyone onto the pavement.' No reply from the swarming people, 'EVERYONE ONTO THE PAVEMENT.'

I was in the middle with a huge smile on my face and my eyes seeing everyone smiling and cheering, wanting a piece of the torch and a photo of me! I felt so proud and so excited and my 'run' hadn't even started yet!

The police cars came first, then some policemen on bikes before a large bus with dancers and musicians and then it was my turn! I saw number 110 walking towards me surrounded by eight security runners who shadowed the torch. He was smiling as he walked towards me then bent over onto one knee as a man would when proposing! We had arranged for him to do this in the bus before his run and it worked perfectly! One of the runners put a stick into my torch to turn the gas on and as the flame bent towards my torch I pushed the head towards it. The gas met with the flame and lit with the reaction of a huge flame coming from my torch and a massive cheer from the crowd! The 'kiss' is the name given when the torches meet and it worked as planned and I was ready to go on and start my run!

A big smile covered my face as I carried the torch! My feet almost felt like they were floating. Everyone in the whole world must have been watching me do my walk. Everyone could see my smile!

'Do you want to run for a bit?' asked one of the guards.

'I have MS. Can I hold onto your arm for balance? Then yeah, for a little bit!' I held his arm with one hand and the torch with the other and we picked up the pace! The cheers kept going and it felt fantastic! Behind me was Adrian carrying a large banner provided by Coca-Cola with my name on it and my mum in her heels who was struggling to keep up but I loved every minute of it!

In total we are allowed to run for approximately 200 metres but my slot was slightly longer because of some safety reason. I didn't complain! I did slow the run to a walk and enjoyed seeing the crowd! In the distance I could see the person wearing 112. We had to do the kiss again before I handed the torch to the helpers on the bus to stop the flame and then I had to sit on the bus and chat with the other torch bearers about their once in a lifetime runs! What an incredible experience and what a wonderful gift I was given! Carrying the Olympic Torch through Liverpool will be one of those amazing things that will bring a smile to my face on any occasion! I was a torch bearer for the London 2012 Olympic Games on 1st June 2012 which was a stunning, sunny day with the majority of my family! Amazing experience, amazing moment, amazing life!

I have been a part of history!

CHAPTER 75
London Paralympic Games, 2012

Conclusion

Four silver medals and one bronze one, more medals than anyone else in Great Britain able or disabled but still a huge disappointment for me. I expected a gold for the 100m Backstroke but obviously I hadn't done enough training, and I wasn't good enough on this occasion. This all sounds very bitter but I was so annoyed believing I could have done better. I suppose the harsh reality check was that everybody wanted to win that gold medal too and that on this occasion someone else wanted it more than me. Looking at it from a more realistic point of view I do have MS; I shouldn't even be in the swimming pool let alone winning numerous medals, but I see the MS as an excuse only! I am defeating the illness and bending the rules which is a wonderful thing for me and for anyone with an illness or ailment of any kind. Fourteen years ago I was struggling to move and praying that I was going to be able to see every time I woke up. I believed that I had done something wrong and that this awful illness was my punishment or my payback, even though I had no idea what it was I had done so incredibly wrong. Hopefully I have now inspired people to believe that an end - for example getting cancer or MS - need not be the actual end of your life.

This book was written originally to tell my family how much I was hurting and explain to them the reasons I kept crying but it is now proof that dreams can stay alive even when they have been crushed, shattered, burned or completely destroyed. Please keep believing in yourself and your dreams can and will come true, eventually! There is a light at the end of the tunnel even if you don't see it yet. A smile paints a thousand pictures but costs nothing to produce. One of your smiles may change everything for the other person you are talking to or walking down the street as they will have to smile in return. Do your good deed of the day and let someone smile too.

Now I will take you on a trip through my London 2012 Paralympics Games Experience!

London Paralympics Games - The greatest show on earth, my home Games with the immense crowd which I feel was the most awe-inspiring part of the Games. My home Games, my home crowd and all that incredible support! This was better than any dream I had ever dreamed.

I was so excited as I packed my bags for the 2012 Paralympics Games, and I felt ready to race my fastest ever races. I had done all the hard training and I had swum the distance. I was ready! The main holding camp for the Paralympics swimmers was held in Manchester. The rest of the Great Britain Paralympics team, however, went to my home town of Bath where they stayed in the university's rooms, apparently. Although these are great they were not quite as luxurious as the rooms in the Hilton Hotel in Manchester which all the Paralympics swimmers were awarded with!

We all went from Manchester to London on a smart Virgin train and everyone was both nervous and excited and ready for their race/s. Arriving in London and seeing the vastness of the Olympic Village only added to my anticipation. Looking around my mouth opened in awe - incredible! There were signs everywhere and security gates, buses… everything! It was so huge that golf buggies with drivers were on hand to transport the athletes around the park's many facilities.

There was one main food hall that the athletes used for their meals. In the food hall, every dish imaginable was served free to the athletes, be they frogs' legs (yuck!) or a McDonald's Big Mac (McDonald's was one of the main sponsors of the Olympics and the Paralympic Games). My favourite meal is lasagna, and there was plenty of Italian lasagna or other pasta to fuel my performance at the Games!

The apartment that I shared with five other athletes seemed to cater for our every wish. It was spacious and there was a lounge where we could socialise and watch Channel 4 TV (another of the main sponsors who covered the whole of the Paralympics Games). We were cut off from all other TV channels and media such as radio, but this only served to increase my anticipation for my races and contact with the watching world. I had to view the opening ceremony for the Paralympics on TV as I was racing within the first three days of the Games. It would have meant too much walking for me should I have had to attend the ceremony itself but I did go to bed that night imagining walking out in front of the audience wearing my GB team kit and a face full of pride!

Unfortunately, I couldn't relax in the lounge with my favourite tipple - a cup of tea - as although our apartment in the Olympic Village had every soft drink imaginable (thanks to Coca-Cola - another amazing sponsor) there were no teabags - I should have brought my own! Adrian brought some for me on a different occasion along with a kettle. We had single beds to sleep in with our very own special Paralympics pillow case and duvet which we obviously brought back home with us afterwards. What lovely memorabilia for the athletes.

To me, this Olympic Village was a kingdom - a kingdom of dreams. Dreams that I, and every other athlete there, had of achieving our very best performance ever. This was a kingdom for the best of the best in every field. The atmosphere in the village pulsated with the athletes' anticipation of competing and achieving our dreams - dreams that years of hard training had created!

Our apartment had patio doors which backed onto the village, and from there we could see the fireworks of the opening ceremony. Each explosion of colour in the night sky seemed to lift my spirits high in anticipation for the races. The atmosphere was electric in this Olympic Village, this kingdom of dreams.

Very close to the Olympic Village was a 1.9 million square foot shopping mall, built especially for the Olympians. Although I didn't have massive amounts of spare time with my family, when we were able to see each other we would walk to the mall and enjoy meals together. In fact, I was incredibly fortunate in the time I had together with my family. Both they and Adrian had rented a house together in Ashford, Kent and they would use the Javelin Train Service especially set up for the Olympics. It would only take thirty minutes for my family to reach London, and with eight super-fast trains running every hour it was very convenient.

It is amusing how little incidents make up the fabric of family fun times. One memory we always laugh about involved an upside-down sheep! In the farm next to the home my family were renting was a flock of sheep. One of the sheep was lying on its back with its legs in the air. My sister Kristy was very worried that the sheep was ill or on its deathbed, despite being assured by the farmer that sheep do in fact lie on their backs sometimes. As the hours passed, the sheep did not turn over, and Kristy is now teased for repeating over and over, 'We've got to save this sheep!'

Kristy was so worried about the sheep that she tried to force Nicholas and Adrian to push it over back on its feet! After an incredible *forty-eight* hours, and because Kristy was pushing them so much, Nicholas and Adrian pushed the sheep over and they all watched as the sheep trotted off back to its flock.

'Yeah! We have saved the sheep!' was Kristy's celebration song!

We still look back and laugh at the funny sheep lying on its back for a full two days, and my family's concern over saving its little life! We filmed the whole event on an iPad so we can watch whenever we need a giggle!

Some of my time at the Olympics was taken up with interviews. In fact, before the Olympics I visited the velodrome for an event organised by Coca-Cola. Westfield shopping mall was also the place where, before the Olympics, all dressed up in my Commonwealth kit, Dizzee Rascal and I did a production. It is wonderful to be able to travel to different locations and meet people from all walks of life. I have been offered some amazing experiences which I am deeply grateful for - incredible chances that most people can only dream about. I am so blessed.

My family and Adrian were a great support to me when I raced. Adrian particularly enjoyed the atmosphere of an eighteen thousand-strong crowd. My first race was 100m Butterfly which I enjoy swimming even though it is so hard. I swam the heats but not in a great time. I qualified for the finals, however, where I came fifth. This was a bit of a shock as I expected to swim really well as I had done all that training.

'Stephanie, 100m Backstroke tomorrow! I hope you enjoy it!' Adrian kissed me good night.

The next day I was excited: 100m Backstroke, my chance at gold, come on girl, you can do it!' The heats were quite good and I qualified for the finals in second place!

For each of the races, the athletes had to walk out from behind a curtain and onto the poolside and this was such a special time because of the crowd's reaction.

'In lane five we have, representing Great Britain, Stephanie Millward!'

'WWWWWAAAAAAAYYYYYYYY!'

The crowd all screamed for me and a huge smile came to my face! 18,000 people were cheering for me, never mind all the people watching on their television sets at home! I felt so good when I got behind the blocks! This was my favorite race.

'Enjoy it,' Adrian had said as had Julia Airlie, my coach from Corsham! 'Enjoy it Stephanie! You are at your very own Olympic/ Paralympics Games and everyone is cheering for you. This is your dream.'

I swam quite well, finishing in second place. I am second in the whole wide world! Second! I was annoyed that I hadn't won the gold but the girl who came first swam faster than my personal best time so on this occasion she therefore deserved to win. After my race I struggled to stand and a couple of people had to help drag me into my wheelchair. They pushed me off poolside so I could get ready for my medal ceremony. I went to the pool for my swim-down then got changed and blow-dried my hair so I looked nice for my presentation.

The Paralympians were given two tracksuits: both in red, white and blue but one with more white which was the one we wore to the races, and one that was more blue which we wore to the presentations. We were also given a pair of fantastic red trainers which I still wear with pride. I changed into my blue tracksuit (the one that everybody recognises) and moved over to the registration area where we had to meet before the medal ceremonies. I was placed in the first spot behind the young ladies who were carrying the medals and behind me was the gold medal winner followed by the third place bronze medal winner. When the music started we walked out onto the poolside then stopped behind the podium. I smiled the whole time, feeling amazing! Because my legs were wobbly after my race I had to ask someone to walk next to me so I could hold their arm to help with my stability. This same person helped me to stand up to the podium when I was called.

'In silver place, from Great Britain, Stephanie Millward!'

I stood up, putting my hand forward to shake the hand of the presenter and accept my bouquet of flowers. The cheer from the crowd was amazing and increased when I put the bouquet of flowers up in the air towards the crowd. The experience shall remain with me forever. The silver medal round my neck was so shiny and so heavy. It weighs approximately half a kilogram! I went for dinner with my family and showed them my medal which they were all so impressed by. What a special dinner, with the people I love, celebrating an unforgettable experience.

After the 100m Backstroke I was given two days off where I didn't have any races - just training - and I used this as a perfect opportunity to do an interview with CBBC. I knew the wonderful presenter, Katie Monaghan, from my school days. Katie is a lovely person but she also struggled with an illness that affects her legs and she often has to rest in her wheelchair. Katie saw this as a wonderful chance for me to be interviewed by a very young boy called Reuben who has Down's syndrome. Reuben was great at talking to me during the interview and he especially loved holding the medal which was on show! This was later shown on the television. What an exciting addition to an already incredible Paralympics.

The press were always standing around waiting to catch everyone for interviews. One person waiting for me was my good friend Oliver Holt (from the Daily Mirror), who always is so supportive. I remember just after the Olympic and Paralympics trials when he came to speak to me. He introduced himself saying that he had taken his two daughters to watch some of the good swimmers but that they had spotted me - perfectly able before my race, with the most powerful yet pretty strokes - yet then I shook viciously afterwards. They had been interested in finding out what was wrong with me so their dad decided to interview me for his article in the Daily Mirror. I told his daughters that we would go swimming together and I hope we will do one day. Oliver Holt - a wonderful man to know.

At another memorable interview in London, just after one of my races, I was afflicted by spasms and one of the reporters wanted to interview me. I was sitting in my wheelchair but I wanted to do the interview standing up! Although you couldn't see them, I had one person holding me around my waist to steady me, one person on each side of me holding onto my arms, and another four ready to help me stand or to catch me if I fell as I was shaking so much!!

I received and still receive a lot of support from my local radio stations. I am good friends with an amazing man called Will Walder and a few of the other incredible BBC Wiltshire radio presenters! They are always cheering me on and often come to all the exciting places that I go to! They are such a support. On one occasion Will Walder gave me a whole tub of gorgeous ice cream. Thank you, Will.

Another great support for me are the local newspapers: the *Gazette*, the *Herald*, the *Wiltshire Times* and, of course, the amazing *Bath Chronicle* (who have been a great support since helping me fight for Betaferon all those years ago). I never felt like I was swimming on my own as I knew I had a strong support team behind me.

My MS affected me at the Games but thankfully there were always kind and helpful people to help me. For example, whenever I swam in a relay I would have to be guided by one of my teammates when I'd finished across the lanes and under the lane ropes. They would be my eyes and would call out to me when the lane was clear so I could make my way across to the side of the pool. It is this thoughtfulness and help that I value, as it gives me a quality of life as well as the ability to participate in my chosen sport. And when I finish a race and hear a 'Congratulations!' from a teammate, I feel as if I've achieved something great as a member of Great Britain's wonderful Paralympic swimming team!

The recurring pain in my left arm was treated through the use of an altitude tent at a local university. Both beforehand and on my days off, I would be driven by the Game's Makers to the university where I would sit inside the altitude tent. There I would either read a book or listen to music. It proves that MS can be managed through the help and support of others, and that dreams can be achieved no matter how great the barrier.

While I was in London I was given a little letter which contained a lovely drawing of me in my GB kit. This was drawn by Nicole, a young girl who suffers from Neurofibromatosis (NF). This is an awful disease which causes Nicole a lot of pain but she still fights her hardest to go to school, and she enjoys doing judo lessons. Nicole and her mum Vanessa came to London to watch and support me, and my family was lucky enough to meet them. I am still trying to go and visit them but chat often over emails. They are an inspirational family.

Security at the Olympics was tight and we were carefully checked upon entering and leaving the Olympic Village. We took specially provided buses to the training and swimming areas, and we had to submit to more security checks when arriving and leaving these locations. There seemed to have been no expense spared with security, the Olympic Village and the training and competing areas! Five Olympic-sized pools had been temporarily built for the athletes to train in. There was also a warm-up/swim-down pool for before and after the races, and of course the all important racing pool! Together, the pools held some ten million liters of water! Amazing! The roof was wave-like in its design and its arena longer than Heathrow's Terminal Five. Wow!

A long time ago I realised I needed to be mentally prepared for each race I swam. I needed to swim each race beforehand in my head, planning each detail down to the finest degree. This I did with my third race which was a 4x100m Freestyle relay. We won bronze for this race. Two silvers followed in the 400m Freestyle and 200m Individual Medley. For the former, a new European record of 4:40 was set! An incredible time for me! I did have an extra battle to fight along with the MS and the spasms and I had a very stiff neck. I just woke up with this stiff neck and I had to go to the physio and let them try to ease the lock that had settled in my neck. The amazing physios, Paul and Ali, had to spend hours trying to release my neck. I swam the 400m Freestyle unable to turn my head to one side and it was so uncomfortable having to breathe on one side only. I wonder how much faster I would have been without the stiff neck which lasted for days.

The last race I was to swim at the Paralympics was the 4x100m Medley Relay. I was to swim the 100m Butterfly and we were hoping for gold as we were the world record holders. Unfortunately the coach we had allocated to us insisted that we leave for the arena, *six hours* prior to the actual race. My teammates spoke up for me, 'Stephanie will never cope without a proper rest for such a long time before the race.'

He did not listen and insisted we left early. As a result we came second missing the gold by three one hundredths of a second behind the winning team from Australia. It was very disappointing and frustrating and we were all near to tears as we knew we should have won that race. I felt that I had lost it because my time had been quite slow. Sitting around at a poolside for six hours exhausts anyone, never mind an MS sufferer where fatigue (intense tiredness) is a key symptom. At least we know we can win it next time as we will be adamant to ignore the coach whatever he says. These are our races and our world records and therefore our gold medals!

The experience at the Games, however, was ultimately a positive one. Little things stood out for me about the 2012 Paralympics races - like a dream where you remember bright colours, heightened feelings and simple words when you wake up. I remember that before stepping out from behind the curtain which separated the swimmers from the racing pool, there was a really cheerful man who would say things to me such as, 'OK, you ready for this race?' and 'You going to swim really fast then?'. He was lovely and always made me smile!

I remember how stepping out from behind the curtain was like stepping out onto a stage. As my name was called - 'Lane four, Great Britain, Stephanie Millward' - the home crowd cheered so loudly. My heart pounded in my chest and I felt like joining in the celebration. I remember the huge noise of support as I stood next to the pool, ready to represent the audience's very own special nation and I remember how it made me want to do my very best!

I remember my striking blue, red and white designer Team GB tracksuit, which I wore when stepping onto the podium to accept my medals. The excitement of the crowd cheering in victory seemed to surge right through me and I remember raising my hand in triumph. The flowing mane of the British lion, etched on the back of all the Paralympian tracksuits, echoed the soaring of my spirits at my victory. I had fought and overcome, as had so many heroes from Great Britain!

Yes, the Paralympics did bring with them disappointments. I did not get the gold in 100m Backstroke and so it was only natural that I felt disappointed in myself. Yet looking at it from a more realistic point of view, I have MS. It is a miracle that I'm even in a swimming pool let alone winning medals! Four silver medals and one bronze - more medals than anyone in Great Britain whether able or disabled.

Adrian said something so important to me after I had won the first medal, 'You have won one silver medal; all you have to do now is enjoy the event.'

So I did! Walking out onto the poolside I had a huge smile on my face and I put up my arm to appreciate the cheer from the crowd! It was incredible. The crowd were incredible! Even the heats were amazing!

'In lane four, from Great Britain, we have Stephanie Millward!'

'YEAH!' Everybody screamed their support and I couldn't help but put my arm up and smile and feel their wonderful support.

'Stephanie you are meant to be getting mentally prepared for your race.'

That cheer from the crowd was all the mental preparation I needed! Thank you!

To Stephanie,

Now over to you. You are a leader of tremendous ability with amazing potential and great, positive ability and you really can achieve all you wish for as long as you don't limit yourself by your external world and internal thought patterns or suggestions that may let you think otherwise.

With so many people saying it couldn't be done, all it takes is an imagination.'
Michael Phelps

'I wouldn't say anything is impossible. I think that everything is possible as long as you put your mind to it and put the work and time into it'.
Michael Phelps

'I concentrate on preparing to swim my race and let the other swimmers think about me, not me about them.'
Amanda Beard

'In most sports they have a physical effect on your performance, in swimming only psychological. If you worry about what your rival is doing, you take your mind off what you are doing and so fail to concentrate on your performance.'

Bacharach, great Chicago coach of the 20s

You can't put a limit on anything. The more you dream, the farther you get'.
Michael Phelps

These quotes come from colleagues of yours in the swimming world, champions just like you are, amazing athletes who went the extra mile, like you do! Challenging the tests of time against the best you can become, like you do! Breaking records that individuals thought were impossible, like you do!

Doing what others don't believe in, like you do! Facing the largest challenges, like you do! Overcoming them, like you do!

GAINING GOLD MEDALS AND BREAKING THE BARRIERS OF TIME, LIKE YOU DOOOOOOO!

So, I hope you enjoyed the read as you truly are a world champion and don't let doubt, fear or anyone take that away from you and do it like you do!

Love,
Andy Milton (My friend forever and my hypnotherapist)

I remember my favourite race - the 100m Backstroke. Every stroke, the turn. I had it all planned out and I remember pushing myself to the utter limit of endurance. And then to finish and to hear I had won silver! I blew a kiss up in the direction of where my family was sitting. Thank you for your amazing support!

I kept remembering Adrian's wise words echoing in my head as I prepared for each race, 'Now that you've won one medal, just go out and enjoy the rest of your races.'

And lastly but probably most importantly, I remember the faces of my family who had travelled from far and wide to see me swim. Paul from New York, Kristy from Columbus, Ohio, Nicholas from Cambodia, my dad from Lincoln and my mum from Lynmouth! As I bent down to accept the heavy silver medal, I remembered their love and support which made this all possible for me. My Adrian, who had motivated me to reach again for my Olympic dream. My mum, a rock and an absolute super star, my angel who had been through every high and low with me. My brothers and sister, my first ever swimming team whose individual successes propelled me forward to achieve this dream. My dad, my hero, whose legacy of love will never leave me. I remember all those who journeyed besides me, and I think, 'We did it! We did it together!'

Please keep believing in yourself, and your dreams can and will come true. There is a light at the end of every tunnel even if you don't see it yet. A smile paints a thousand pictures but costs absolutely nothing to produce. One of your smiles may change everything for someone else as they will have to smile in return. Do your good deed for the day, and let someone smile too.

This chapter about my experience at the London 2012 Paralympics Games is my smile, my gift to you.

CHAPTER 76

My Wonderful Mum!

She is the most inspiring person I have ever met and she amazingly seems to know everything – she is my mum, Ms Linda Millward. Born in Wigan, UK, she was daughter to my nan, Mrs Rita Waite. My Nan was an innocent mother but was not very effective in a family role and when my mum's father decided to do everything he wanted without even thinking of helping my nan, she had no means to fight. My mum saw that her mum had to work to get some money for the family and so she therefore took on the role of mother to her two sisters and one brother. At a very young age she was busy cooking meals, packing lunches and taking the kids to school. My mum was the foster mother or carer for her sisters and brother. My mum went on to marry my dad, Mr Christopher Michael Millward when she was twenty-two, give birth to Paul at the age of twenty-three, me at twenty-five, Kristy at twenty-seven and then Nicholas at twenty-nine. In Jeddah she rode us to playgroup, kindergarten, brownies, tap dancing etc on the back of a four-seated push bike! In that tremendous heat and carrying three of us on the bike I am sure it was very hard work. Paul, thankfully, was able to ride his own bike! My mum learned a lot from her experiences and this is why I had such a perfect life. My mum never got the chance to go to ballet lessons so she took Kristy and me to ballet and brownies and tap dancing, horse riding, roller skating, ice skating and swimming. She offered us everything and I will be forever grateful. My mum has basically offered her children everything that she used to dream about as a child. We were living her dreams. My mum never did as well at school as she probably should have done but only because she was so busy trying to be the mother of the family. If she was to do a degree now I am certain she would be awarded a first because of her determination, her complete understanding of life, knowledge and her natural common sense.

My mum even brought her children up without the thrill of sweets as a treat. While in Saudi Arabia we ate only apples as a desert and sometimes had ice cream when we went to warm places on holiday. Because of having no introduction to sweets I never wanted or needed them. This has been very good for my teeth because as I do not tend to eat sweet thing. My teeth are very strong and good and I do not have any fillings! All thanks to my mum!

When I first got MS I pushed everyone away, spending most of my time in my room with Spring. Whenever I came out for work or for my main meals my mum would be the first to ask me how I felt and to see me smile through my tear-ridden eyes. When I went blind my mum was the strength by my side keeping me looking up, keeping me hoping for the future. When Spring died it was my mum who looked for and found a second guardian angel, a second Yorkshire terrier, Maisie, who again spent most of her time by my side. When I failed my exams it was my mum who kept reminding me that I had been chosen as one of the brightest eight in the year to go to a special maths class every Saturday morning at Bath University. It was my mum who reminded me that almost nobody passes their driving test first time especially when you have to ruin your chances straight away by telling the examiner that you have Multiple Sclerosis. It was my mum who arranged for my injections to be sent to me when I was in Australia and again on holiday with Kristy. It was my mum who had to fight her own fears and learn to inject her daughter, to cause more pain to someone you love. I probably won't have a child of my own and that is because I don't believe I can be a good enough mum. My mum was perfect and she did and still does everything for me whenever I need help. In her place I think I would have run away. I don't think I could have been even nearly as strong as her. My mum should be commended for all the support she has given to me and the rest of her family. She is a wonderful person and even more than that she is a wonderful mother. She is an angel in disguise and she has been perfect in my fight for life. With my mum by my side we are always going to be the winners. I believe that I can do anything now even with the MS and that now all the barriers have been raised. My mum is someone very special to me and I hope everything in her life goes as planned. Mummy, I love you more than life itself. You are my strength, my sun, my hope! Thank you, mum, for being my wonderful mum! I couldn't have dreamed of anyone better! You are amazing in every single way!

CHAPTER 77
Freedom of Corsham!

Freedom of Corsham - what an honour! I felt so special that I had been awarded such an incredible award. Apparently the only people who have ever been awarded this before were in the army and now I was the first individual person to be awarded the Freedom of Corsham! AMAZING!

The celebration was wonderful with it all starting at the Methuen Arms pub which is situated at one end of the high street in Corsham. Here I did an interview with BBC Wiltshire radio and the wonderful presenter, Will Walder. A few of the local papers were there taking pictures and I felt so happy and so excited!

After the interviews I put all my five medals won in London 2012 around my neck with each medal weighing half a kilogram so my poor neck struggled with the weight but the adrenaline from the day allowed me to fight the pains! I gave my Olympic Torch to one of the swimmers who trained with Corsham ASC (my home club). I walked out of the Methuen Arms to be greeted by hundreds of children who had come to Corsham town especially for the celebration! It was amazing. I showed off the medals and chatted to all the children and their parents! The incredible Corsham Band were playing some lovely tunes and I was asked to start walking up the high street so I did, with all these people also following me! I was smiling the whole way! When we eventually got to the Town Hall which is placed at the other end of the High Street there were even more people waiting for my arrival, all with smiles on their faces! The local butcher had invited me into his shop before to taste different flavours of sausage so that we could choose the best one to be named after me for my day! They decided to sell a specially made Stephanie Millward sausage which was korma flavoured! I loved the taste even though I never eat sausages normally! The Stephanie Millward sausages were on sale for everyone to buy!

A number of schools had produced dances as a way of supporting me and my Freedom of Corsham day and so they did their production in front of me, the Mayor and some councillors! I was definitely touched by what everyone was doing! One of the dances spelt out my name which was incredible. There were personalised balloons and Union Jacks everywhere and people had put all sorts of posters in their shops celebrating my special day! The whole town bent over backwards to make me feel special and I felt the love from everyone which was such a powerful feeling, one I will never forget!

My friend and wonderful hairdresser, Natalie Brown, had made me look really pretty that morning so I felt good! I was surrounded by all my amazing friends! I had the time of my life!! The own Mayor did a lovely speech in front of the crowd outside of the Town Hall and I did a little speech too feeling brilliant! I was given a huge bouquet of flowers from a town councillor and another from Pak who owns the local Chinese and who is an amazing support of mine! Pak has a picture of him and me up in his Chinese for everyone to see! He is so proud of the things I have done!

After the speeches I tried to go around everyone and speak to them all thanking them for coming and signing autographs! I love writing a few inspiring words for everyone. Hopefully something I have said will help someone to do something they never thought possible! I had been asked to name twenty to twenty-five special friends that would get invites into the Town Hall for Champagne and some snacks! This was so hard because I wanted everyone to be a part of the day. I needed Adrian's help to cut the list down to twenty-five! These twenty-five people were invited into the Town Hall where we all had seats. The head coach from Corsham ASC and a good friend of mine, Julia Airlie, did a gorgeous speech standing on the stage and everyone listened with smiles on their faces! The Mayor also did a speech about this special day and awarded me with a salver. Adrian and I had to sign a book which will be kept for anyone to see in the future! My parents both looked so proud of me! I am glad I helped to give them a special day too! What an amazing experience! A wonderful day, in a wonderful town, full of wonderful people! Amazing!

CHAPTER 78

Planning the Wedding

For our amazing, wonderful, incredible, dream white wedding Adrian and I spent a lot of time looking through hotels trying to find the perfect one. It had to be a special place worthy of the love and life I was to give to Adrian. We wanted everyone to feel the love we share.

We wanted it to happen close to our home (Corsham, Wiltshire) so we started there and I asked my mum to look too. We went for Bryers House and another mansion but my mum came up with Bailbrook House. Adrian and I went to the Castle Combe Manor House and watched as a bride was having photos with her husband and her guests. We then went inside to look through the building. It felt like we were given a good price for what it was offering but it just didn't feel right. The Combe Down golf club looked good too, very friendly and the organiser was informative but something important was missing. Adrian had been to these venues many times before while playing golf so this made these venues incorrect for us. Mum's choice of Bailbrook House proved to be the one and only perfect place for our wedding. It is in Batheaston which is close to the church we were going to use which was in Box the area I love after living there for twelve years! It is also close to where the majority of my friends live which makes it easy for everyone! I am so excited about this and hopefully our wedding will be perfect for us!

The planning started with me looking on the internet to get a list of things we needed to do. Mum as always helped by informing me of all the things the internet didn't advise! A save-the-date card was first on the list but I needed to do the guest list even before that. My guest list was an incredible length and I realised that I might not be able to invite everyone and that I had to be a bit more selective so my list of 300 had to be halved even before I added Adrian's side of the family! This was a bit of a nightmare for me but I had to think about the total cost of the wedding!

The wedding was completely organised and we felt that everything was going to be perfect! Unfortunately, though, things are never that easy! Bailbrook House was bought by a new owner and they said that they would have to cancel a number of weddings as the venue would be a bit of a building site. Colin Bush (a very good friend of mine) came with me to the hotel to see which parts we were going to be allowed to use. It seemed OK but I was very annoyed that the plans had changed so much. In the end we weren't able to use Bailbrook House at all and they offered us a couple of other options so we went to visit these sites but unfortunately neither was perfect. Four months before our wedding date we were frantically searching for an available wedding venue. Truthfully it was always right in front of our eyes! On my way to school every day I had passed it and every time I drove from Box to Corsham or Chippenham I passed it! Why I hadn't thought of it before I don't know but it was perfect, well kind of! Adrian, my mum and I went into Rudloe Hall Hotel to meet the wedding organiser who was very nice. She showed us round the venue and told us their prices. It wasn't too expensive and seemed to have everything we wanted. Bailbrook House offered us some compensation because they had cancelled at such late notice. I had to produce a spreadsheet showing the costs of everything we had ordered at Bailbrook with their prices in comparison to the prices for the same thing in Rudloe Hall hotel. In the end Bailbrook House gave us compensation which definitely helped.

My mum, while doing a good job at being our wedding planner, noticed all the things wrong, old or tired at the site at Rudloe Hall hotel: the damp on the ceiling; the broken tiles; the spiders' webs;

the bad carpets that needed carpet grips to make it easier and safer to walk across. I knew we had invited guests who might bring their wheelchairs or sticks so we needed it to be easy for them. I sent the hotel wedding planner a list of things we wanted to be changed for our wedding such as repaint lots of areas and we wanted the grounds to be safe to walk on! The road up to the hotel was very bumpy so I asked for this to be gravelled or to get rid of all the pot holes. Adrian's best man, Matthew Leighton-Fry, arranged it so he could get the pot holes filled if necessary on the morning of the wedding! He was amazing saying he would get the list sorted if the hotel didn't do it themselves. This was so comforting to hear! This hotel had just been taken over by Marco Pierre White and I didn't have anything to worry about! The hotel built a disabled toilet which was incredibly useful for the guests and they did everything my list had asked for. Just before the wedding when we visited the site we were amazed with the changes - incredible!

The night before the wedding my sister and I stayed in a room in the hotel and my mum helped us organise the freshly varnished and painted function room. We put the candles in their places and the hotel wedding planner was amazing helping us to do everything. We felt so relaxed and so happy! Lights were put up everywhere and we had big jars full of pink penny sweets, a pretty white wishing tree ready for the good luck messages and an antique brown leather miniature suitcase for the wedding cards. Everything was perfectly in place for tomorrow. Everyone went back to their homes or their hotels and Kristy and I went back to our room to rest ready for tomorrow, one of the biggest days of my life!

Adrian McHugh to marry Stephanie Millward. When two become one!

CHAPTER 79
Our Wedding

Adrian and his best man, Matt Leighton-Fry, and the ushers, my brothers Paul and Nicholas, and Adrian's sister Alison's sons Tyrone and Tyson Pollard got to the church very early all preparing for the ceremony! The vicar was there also making sure that everything was just the way it was supposed to be! The organist was there too enjoying his job and loving the smiles and the friendly banter from all the guests! The choir was excited and everyone who walked into the church commented on how pretty it was.

My mum, Kristy and I were busy trying to get every photo perfect and every strand of hair in the right place! My dad opened a bottle of Champagne which we obviously enjoyed after the toast made by my dad! Coming down the stairs with a huge smile on my face I heard a neigh from outside the hotel; my horse and carriage were waiting patiently for me to arrive! We had ordered two white shire-type horses with a gorgeous white carriage and I got into the carriage with my dad ready for the ride to the church! Paul Langley, a good friend of mine, after giving me a hug and kiss on my cheek drove a stunning Rolls Royce that Kristy and my mum were overjoyed with getting to sit in! We all got to the church fashionably late! There were some friends outside of the church wishing me well and wanting me to smile for the cameras! The local paper was there too which I was pleased to see! Eventually, my mum went into the church following the vicar and this is when the music changed and Adrian realised that I must have arrived! I had told him about the tape that would play just before I entered and he stood up with Matt ready for the next change of song.

'Do not turn around until Stephanie enters the church,' Adrian was told about two or three times by the vicar before Adrian turned the correct way!

'Here Comes the Bride' started being played by the organist and a smile crept onto both of our faces! My dad and I started walking forward in time to the music. 'Walk slowly and enjoy every second' my dad had said so we did. I looked around but couldn't see anything for a bit because it had been so light outside and therefore so dark relatively inside. This made me giggle! I saw a number of my friends in the church and the families as I moved up the aisle. Amazing they were all here for our special day!

Bang! I hit one of the lit candles that Matt and the ushers had placed in the aisle to light my path! The glass lantern fell to the ground but I kept moving and Sarah Leighton-Fry kindly picked up the lantern and placed it back in its place!

My dad and I walked up to our positions in the church and I was met by Adrian who looked very handsome. Matt was stood by his side also looking very proud! Kristy pulled up next to me and started arranging my veil and headpiece and the flowers were thrown to my dad to hold for a moment! Once I looked good Kristy moved over with my dad and the ceremony was ready to begin.

The vicar welcomed us in to the church. We had done a rehearsal a couple of days ago so we were ready for all the exciting speeches. Adrian and I had asked Alastair Hignell, Paul, Nicholas and Heather Marshall to do readings for us. Alastair was the first one and he read a lovely poem that made me smile! Nicholas was the second after we had sang one of our hymns. Nicholas gave a lovely reading about love which I really enjoyed and then Paul was the next one and he read Corrintheus 21, a reading from the Bible. It was a perfect reading and he did it very well indeed. The vicar kept on commenting on Paul's reading as it was a good reference to the love between Adrian and I which was being honoured and celebrated today! The next speaker was Heather Marshall who did a lovely reading for us! Heather read from *Captain Corelli's Mandolin*.

Love is a temporary madness, it erupts like volcanoes and then subsides. And when it subsides you have to make a decision. You have to work out whether your root was so entwined together that it is inconceivable that you should ever part. Because this is what love is.

Love is not breathlessness, it is not excitement, it is not the promulgation of promises of external passion. That is just being in love, which any fool can do. Love itself is what is left over when being in love has burned away, and this is both an art and a fortunate accident.

Those that truly love have roots that grow towards each other underground, and when all the pretty blossoms have fallen from their branches, they find that they are one tree and not two.

From *Captain Corelli's Mandolin* by Louis de Bernières

I love this quote and it was amazing that Heather read it so well. After Heather's words it was time for Adrian and I to make our own vows. Adrian and I have watched and enjoyed all of the series of Smallville which is a series about Superman and of his true, love Lois Lane. Adrian and I watched their wedding in the series and used their words to help write our own vows!

Our vows:

Stephanie: I wanted these vows to be perfect, but perfection is a hard thing to get your hands on

But life is meant to be a little messy and when it comes to love you only sign up for it if it is the only thing you can ever imagine doing.

Adrian: I Adrian McHugh take you Stephanie Millward to be my companion, for ever, with you by my side I will never be alone.

Stephanie: You are my best friend, you are my hope, you are my true love and I am yours and will be forever.

Adrian: On this day, at this moment, I pledge the rest of my life to you.

You've always believed in me and I believe in you and when you believe in someone it is not for a minute, not just for a second, it is forever.

After our lovely vows the vicar continued with the normal vows. Adrian and I looked lovingly into each other's eyes as we both said 'I do'!

Our wedding was full of love and the choir helped to make perfect music! Leaving the church at the end of the ceremony I felt truly loved by all my friends and family! Towards the end of the ceremony when we were signing the legal papers a young girl called Zara sang a lovely song for us; she was amazing and everyone listened with open mouths. What an incredible singer!

Adrian and I stood outside of the church covered by the sunshine as all our guests came out of the church. It was amazing to speak to everyone and they all said how much they loved the wedding! Lots of photos followed from the newspapers and from our friends and family! The next step was walking up to the horses and the carriage and all our guests threw confetti over us! It was a lovely feeling walking through all our smiling, happy friends after our amazing wedding!

We got into the carriage and the horses had to canter to get some of the way up the steep hill. Sorry guys! We had three breaks on our ride to the hotel because both the horses were ready for retirement and this was their last ever ride. I loved the breaks as I sat in the carriage with a massive smile on my face loving everything about the day! Two horses in an adjoining field cantered by the fence to try to be part of our herd! It was lovely to see those horses joining in on our fantastic day! Alison, Adrian's sister, who was so excited and happy about the day, saw us having a break and was desperate to beep the cars horn before Dale reminded her that the horses would probably hate the sound of the horn and might have been spooked by it. I am glad Dale jumped in there!

Adrian and I got to the hotel quite late but still received a massive cheer from all our waiting guests! Victoria Klewin was singing lovely songs for us and we listened with amazement at the sound of her stunning voice! The function room looked absolutely beautiful with all of the flowers that were on the tables and all the lighting! It all looked so amazing and everyone had a huge smile on their faces! We sat down at the top table which had Joan McHugh, John McHugh (Adrian's dad), Matt Leighton-Fry, Adrian, me(!), my mum, Linda Millward, Kristy Millward, and my dad, Mike Millward. Adrian lost his mum, Jane, to cancer when he was just twenty-one, but in some way I hope she was watching her son get married to me and I hope she feels very proud of him!

The food was brilliant with leek and potato soup as the starter, beef bourguignon with mashed potato and vegetables for the main meal then a fantastic chocolate cake, which I could have eaten thousands of if I had the choice! It was an amazing meal! Afterwards it was time for the speeches with Matt being the compere telling everyone when to speak. My dad was the first to speak and his was a lovely speech although the tears forced him to finish early. He sounded so proud of me. We have all been through so much and travelled so far and dad just couldn't control his emotions. I was amazed that I could, truthfully, as tears are never far from my eyes normally. My mum was the next speaker and normally mums don't speak at a wedding but when I got sick my mum was my life and soul and she was the person helping me to pick up my broken jigsaw puzzle and who dried my eyes when the emotions just flooded out. My mum's speech was amazing. We almost lost nan last year and I remember sitting at the hospital bed wondering how we could bring this lifeless body back to life. Her coma calmed down and just before we were going to turn off her life support we saw a flicker of her eyelids - this was enough. Paul flew back from America, saw the body lying there and couldn't understand why we were saying she was much better that day! Mum had to applaud nan for being able to come to the wedding after her fight with the coma. Matt, the best man, was the next speaker and he did what best men do and knocked Adrian down a couple of times but made us all laugh madly! Adrian's speech was last. Adrian thanked everyone for coming and he thanked Paul and Kerry, Paul's partner for paying for the wedding cake. He then started off with an amazing speech that made everyone laugh uncontrollably about our fight with Sat Nav! We never seem to be able to get anywhere without having a problem with Sat Nav or closed roads and as usual we have to phone my mum for help! It was so funny because it happens so often!

Everyone was in a great mood when we moved to another room for the tables to be cleared and the room to be changed into a dance floor. This room had the wedding cake in it which was stunning with huge icing roses on the side! The cake had been made by Robyn Seviour and it was amazing!

When the dance floor was opened we all moved in ready for a dance! The first dance was our first dance and we had chosen Snow Patrol's 'Chasing Cars' which has been a favourite of ours for a long time. The second dance was for me and my dad. I had chosen Tim McGraw's 'My Little Girl' because I love the song and it seemed perfect! After these two songs everyone joined in the dancing! We had such an amazing evening full of fun and excitement! We had a wedding perfect for our dreams! I am living that fairytale life with the perfect husband, perfect life and perfect friends! Everything is perfect now, a life to be so very proud of!

A life, my life, full of dreams that have all come true!

CHAPTER 80

Aquae Sulis

One hundred children, lanes packed full of people, lots of noise, no Great Britain costumes – why on earth did I chose Aquae Sulis instead of the ITC (Intensive Training Centre) where I would have been able to train with approximately only eight other swimmers? Why did I make this strange choice? Firstly I wanted someone to race and in a lane where I would have been just about on my own I would have raced only myself, but in a lane full of young teenagers with growing egos desperate to be the best and certain they can beat you whatever stroke they do I definitely would have someone to race! Secondly, I chose Aquae Sulis because I had no other option. Because I had a disability I was obviously not right to train with any of the able-bodied swimmers as a part of the ITC Team Bath group. They didn't need or want me slowing them down which was a shame really. So my options were stay at Swansea miles away from the man I was going to marry or choose a local club like Aquae Sulis. Aquae Sulis is made up of a number of swimmers from around Wiltshire and BANES who have swam very well at their county events and are seen as the best swimmers in the area. A number of national qualifying swimming times are met every year by the swimmers which make the team an amazing selection of brilliant swimmers and very determined young people! I did think maybe the coach wouldn't be good enough but after meeting Martin Mosey and watching how he interacted with the children and knowing that a coach doesn't necessarily always make a good swimmer I knew Aquae Sulis was right for me. 'Aquae Sulis', what a strange name. So I looked it up on Wikipedia: Aquae Sulis was a small town in the Roman Province of Britannia. Today it is known as Bath, located in the English county of Somerset. An obvious name for the team!

Martin Mosey was a wonderful coach pushing us all on when we were swimming slow and congratulating when swimming fast! Martin came to Sheffield to watch me swim a few times and I felt very proud that he had come all that way just for me! Martin helped me win my four golds and one silver at the World Championships in Canada and so I will always be grateful of him! Unfortunately, as people do, some individuals thought the grass was greener on the other side of the fence or, in this case, with a different coach so they make a complaint regarding the aggressiveness of the way Martin spoke to children when they were messing around. Truthfully, I didn't think he was doing anything more than a teacher would or should do. Martin had to go through tribunals, have his teaching licence taken from him and was sent away from the squad he had happily built up over a number of years. I will always think of Martin Mosey as the guy who helped me win those World Championship medals and never as a tyrant in any way. Good luck Martin!

British Swimming stepped in to help find a coach for Aquae Sulis and they knew of a perfect person - John Dougall. John had been a swimmer himself competing at international level and doing well at just about all the strokes! John came to Aquae Sulis and noticed our awful almost lazy turns straight away so he set off immediately working on the turns and kicks. With MS my legs have taken a beating and prove to be a lot weaker than before. John thinks highly of strengthening the legs so that they can work hard during the whole race and the arms would just be added on top. This is great except when my legs start screaming at me after the first length of kick! Pain is all in the mind, I kept telling myself, it is not real. So I pushed my legs as hard as they would go. After a kick set I struggled to walk and would often have to have someone help me get out of the pool after a very hard session. John is a nice coach who likes to work us hard and see all the bright red faces during the training session but he also dislikes the children messing around and will send the swimmers out to get changed if they don't stop talking or answer back or if they are just being lazy! He likes everyone working hard on the technique parts of the stroke and I agree that this is the most important part of any stroke. When I was younger I always made sure my stroke technique was as near to perfect as I could get it which helped when I came back to swimming eventually because the strokes were already there and all I needed was to get fit again!

There were a few swimmers who have helped me so much since I started with Aquae Sulis. They are all very special individuals and I am very proud to know them! First one is Flo. Florence Legg is a backstroke swimmer through and through! She has been swimming for what seems like forever, she says, starting when she was very young and has been going to national competitions since the age of fourteen! Flo is very clever and is planning on going to university originally to train to become a GP but now has changed it to a clinical engineer! Amazing, clever, young lady. Whenever my eyesight gets dizzy or I find it difficult to see after a hard set I sit just behind Flo in the lane and wait for her double kick when she turns for her tumble turn. When I feel the double kick I know it is almost time for my turn and therefore my double kick! Flo is my eyes when I need her help! Flo always will bend over backwards to help! She is a lovely, incredible person and I am so glad I have her as a good friend!

Sophie Minnican, an accountant-to-be, an impressive freestyle swimmer with more opinions than anyone I know! If we want to say something to the coach or if we are not happy with the session plan just tell Sophie and she will tell the coach and everyone else actually for us which is a great idea! I love the way she is so loud when she needs to be! Sophie was the first person to talk to me when I started training with Aquae Sulis and I am still good friends with her as she is great company! Sophie is a great person and everyone loves her!

Emily Codd started swimming when she was twelve years old but two years later she qualified to compete in the Irish Nationals in freestyle, butterfly and an individual medley event. Emily has got an incredible kick so when you are following her you can see nothing but a whole pool full of bubbles. She is an amazing swimmer and a lovely very positive person! After what seems like a very slow warm-up Emily shoots in front and races the rest of the session! She always brings a smile to my face! SPEEDY!

Racheal Wilson (not a typing error for her name!) was home-schooled which I found very interesting and she swims because she loves it. Racheal never misses a session and generally swims at the back of the lane ready for her chance to swim breaststroke, her love! Racheal was point two of a second off her national time this year but I am sure she will get it next year!

Jessie Foster is an amazing swimmer. I had to include her in this book because she amazes me! During one of our 200m Medley sessions Jessie swam a time that was faster than my PB! Wow! Jessie started qualifying for the Nationals when she was just eleven years old and Jessie is also mainly a breaststroke swimmer although obviously very good at medleys too! For 2014 she has qualified for five races at this year's Nationals! This is very good in anyone's eyes! Jessie is a wonderful swimmer.

The leader of the pack is a guy called Alex Keen. Alex is a lovely person always smiling, always happy, always very motivational. I often think of Alex as a black stallion in charge of his herd of mares. On Wednesday mornings we generally have a hard flat out (max) set and Alex always moves lanes to swim in the same lane as me where he takes to the front to show the lane how to do it! He always makes me smile! What a lovely guy!

Seeing all of these incredibly inspirational people surrounding me nine times a week it's no wonder I still have this desire to be the best I can be! Another swimmer who amazes me is a tiny fourteen-year-old boy called Henry Dixon who John has nicknamed Enrie because we have a couple of Henrys in the squad! Enrie is so cute and I always want to buy him a McDonald's to help feed him up and make him grow! I am not sure this would work but it might! Enrie is a 1500m Freestyle specialist because he just keeps going but is very good at butterfly and has qualified for the Nationals on the 1500m and the 400m Freestyle! He will be amazing when he grows a bit!

The other Henry, Henry Clifford, is a lovely person always asking me if he can help in some way! A lovely amazing guy who I am sure will go far in life! Henry is a brilliant swimmer but also the most sincere twitter friend who always sends me really inspiring brilliant tweets that make me smile and feel proud. A lovely person and hopefully a friend for life!

Another couple to mention are Tweedle Dum and Tweedle Dee, Chloe Flower (butterfly) and Becky Hawkins (breaststroke) who giggle one hundred percent of the time and make even the dullest set that bit more exciting!

All of these swimmers are great but there is one boy who helped me immensely on a Friday morning at the Aquaterra pool in the centre of Bath. We had all turned up to training as per usual with the majority of the swimmers still half-way through a REM (rapid eye movement) cycle of sleep. I put my foot into the water to feel the temperature and was shocked at how hot it was. The pool was 36 degrees which is very similar to that of a bath. Oh no I know I struggle with heat especially baths so generally just have showers as baths give me an uncomfortable side effect.

'John I never have a bath because it makes me very dizzy,' I said. 'I might take this session a bit easier.'

'No problem' John replied, trusting that I knew best with the MS.

We all started the session and when we stopped the excited chatter started: 'It is roasting', 'It feels like a bath', 'When you push off the wall in the shallow end there is a tiny bit of cooler water, maybe it will cool the pool down?'. The pool was very hot and although there was a filter that was trying to cool the pool down it didn't work quickly enough! I had to sit on the side of the pool to cool down on quite a few occasions and John realised how bad these swimming conditions were and allowed us to get out early. The only problem was that I was sat on the floor unable to get up as my legs weren't quite over the heat. Here is where my wonderful helper came in! Ben Lawton, my breaststroke friend, put his hand out for me to hold onto to try to get me up! Ben is someone with whom I race a lot during training with him on breaststroke and me on backstroke; although I should win sometimes he is faster which makes me work harder to try to beat him! Ben has always been very positive asking me how I was when we were in training so now he helped me walk to the changing room with Racheal Wilson on my other side with her arm around my waist! They were an amazing team – thank you so much Ben and Racheal! A lot of people I normally chat to at these Aquaterra training session (members of the general public in for their swim too) were worried about me.

'What have you done to your leg?' they asked.

'Nothing it is just my MS, it will be fine again soon!'

Thank you Ben and Rachael for helping me, you have hearts of pure gold!

Another person I need to mention is Tom Sinclair. He is a silent person who turns up to training just to swim. He will answer people's questions but generally won't start any conversations as he is here to train and not to chat. During one of our training sessions he broke one of his fingers and had to stay out of the water for three weeks but on his return swam a 100m Freestyle race with fins on in 51 seconds - amazing!! This is an incredible time especially when he has been out of training for so long with the broken finger! Incredible!

Last but not least is Charlie Head who is a 400m Individual Medley specialist. Charlie is a lovely person who did a speech at school and a presentation about me and the inspiration I have given to him through my fights in life and my swimming. Charlie got an A grade for this speech and he was so proud he told me all about it! I was impressed so when Bath University asked me to meet HRH Prince Edward I invited Charlie to help me with my medals. Charlie obviously agreed with open arms and it was an experience I am certain we will never forget! I will tell you more about that in a later chapter!

Aquae Sulis seems to be a perfect club to train with and the coaches here are amazing with John Dougall in charge of the whole squad, with assistant coaches Andrew Turner, Ritchie and Chrissie Lamb and Mark Harrison all in charge of the age group squads or the main squad when John is away. Andrew Turner is an amazing man. Whenever I am struggling in any way he is always there pushing me on! On the walk back to my car it is Andrew who sees the tired legs struggling and slight limping and always says something very motivating to keep me positive and strong! Thank you so much, Andrew! Ritchie and Chrissie Lamb have a daughter who swims with Aquae Sulis and they are so strong, always there if the help is needed! Amazing people. Mark Harrison tried his hardest to be at the sessions when John was away but he also had to be at his wedding getting married to the love of his life and going on their honeymoon. Mark is one of those people who can be in at least two places at once! A real support! Jamie Forrest, the coach for Bradford on Avon ASC, helps a lot too as he has the knowledge and experience which is very useful for us!

We had a bit of a dilemma at the beginning of 2013 when BANES said that they were going to take away our funding of £40,000 a year. This hit us quite hard and we are still trying to find sponsorship support from anyone. We have done loads of fundraising events trying to keep the club going! The parents again have been amazing! Another issue at the beginning of 2014 was that John Dougall had to have an emergency operation and therefore couldn't coach because he was in hospital and then recovering. The parents and the other coaches tried their hardest to make sure that all the training sessions were still available for the swimmers. It was amazing just how hard everyone tried to keep the club alive! Just in case these two issues weren't enough we have been told that Bath University are going to have to close the pool (the place where we train) for twenty weeks for urgent repairs! Blimey is it me or has this club been hit by a lot of bad luck? Even so all the swimmers come to swimming with huge smiles on their faces all eager to please whichever coach it may be on that day!!

Welcome to my wonderful club, Aquae Sulis! I am so proud to be a part of such an amazing team with all its incredible members!

CHAPTER 81

World Championships, Montreal, 2013

Montreal, Canada, the venue for the IPC World Championships 2013. I went to Canada with a smile on my face and dreams buzzing in my mind! Stephanie Millward, World Champion! Just imagine! That would be amazing! I had never been to Canada before so that was another tick on my places visited list which was exciting! The pool was only a short trip from the hotel and we travelled there by mini buses that the British Swimming staff members drove. The racing pool was very good. Basically the site had two outdoor pools but after the thunder and lightning storms we had in Rio we now have to race in indoor or covered pools. On this occasion they covered one of the pools in a large tent which worked perfectly. The other pool they left open for our warm-up or swim-down sessions.

We arrived in Canada and trained for a couple of days before the event started and it was so exciting seeing other competitors from different countries! I was feeling confident because I had done some good training with my coach, Martin Mosey, and I felt very strong. My first race was 100m Freestyle which has never been one of my best events but I knew I was good at it! I hadn't been allowed to swim this in London because I had apparently too many races already! The heats were very exciting as it was my first race in the competition and

I went to the call-up room with my headphones and my wheelchair (for after the race!). I went through the race in my head then knew I was ready for it! I swam the heats and went into the final in second place and I was very excited about the final later that day! The final for the 100m Freestyle came and I won the gold medal by half a second! Amazing! I just kept on going and nobody came with me! The time wasn't good but that didn't really matter as I had won the gold medal; I was world champion! Being world champion kept making me think about R. Kelly's song 'The World's Greatest'. I love this song as I have always wanted to be the World's Greatest but never really believed that I could be! This is now proof that you can achieve anything if you just believe it enough! I can now sing that song knowing that I am the World's Greatest! What an amazing feeling!

The weather for the whole event was warm and lovely and generally very hot but then we started experiencing huge thunder and lightning storms which meant that we weren't allowed to swim in the outside pool. This ultimately meant that it stopped me from being able to complete any swim-downs which for me are necessary for my walking purposes! After the 100m Freestyle I felt more confident and as part of the relay teams we won the 4x100m Freestyle final and the 4x100m Medley final with me swimming the backstroke leg! I also won the heats of my favourite event, the 100m Backstroke, and the final! The only one of my races I didn't win was the 200m Individual Medley where the swimmer does one length (50m) of butterfly followed by one length of backstroke, then breaststroke and then finishes with one length of front crawl. My breaststroke is my weakest length but after the Paralympics in London where I had come second I knew I was quite good at this race! My 200m IM was good enough to put me second into the final but then the girl who had come first was disqualified! Perfect! I was going into the final in first place! But then, for whatever strange reason, the people in charge of the GB team fought with the volunteer helper who witnessed the girl who had been disqualified and they concluded that they must have made a mistake. For anybody a disqualification is a disqualification irrelevant of your age, sex or stature and I believe this girl should never have been allowed back to swim in the final. I was always taught you have to learn from your mistakes.

On a couple of occasions after racing we were told to go and do interviews for Channel 4 which ended up with me anxious to stand for my interviews with the MS dragging me down. In a number of interviews I had somebody grasping my waist holding me vertical, people on both sides trying to stop the shaking from my spasms and somebody else holding my legs stable! Always have that smile on my face! MS is fighting to be in charge but this is my dream; it has taken it once so never again. I am the winner. I am in control even with my four helpers. I am in charge! Me 1, MS 0.

I won four golds and one silver medal at these World Championships! I am the world champion even with the MS!

World Champion! Is the next step a Paralympic GOLD medal?!

CHAPTER 82

Duke of Edinburgh Awards

The Duke of Edinburgh Awards is a leading youth charity where the Duke of Edinburgh gives all young people aged fourteen to twenty-four the chance to develop skills for life and work, fulfil their potential and have a brighter future.

Well, my gosh, where do I start? I get quite a lot of emails and letters asking me to open fetes, to do speeches at schools or for businesses but when I received a letter stamped HRH I wa as excited as anyone else would be! The letter that I received said that the Duke of Edinburgh would like me (yes, me) to help him award the gold awards for the Duke of Edinburgh gold award winners at St James's Palace in London! Oh, my gosh! What an honour!

I quickly arranged train tickets for Adrian and me to get to London ready for our exciting presentation. I was asked to take all my recent medals and the Olympic Torch which I was thankful of because obviously ten medals for the London Paralympic Games and the Montreal World Championships is quite an accomplishment, never mind the stunning Olympic Torch which always makes me smile! Poor Adrian had to carry the bag though and I am certain his painful shoulders complained for weeks! We were asked to meet at a certain entrance at a particular time where we would be met by a young lady who would then asked me to do a two to three minute interview for the Duke of Edinburgh's website. As we waited by the gates I did stand out a bit in my London 2012 GB kit but this didn't really matter as I felt so proud of myself! It is great to be noticed and still amazing how much attention the London Stella McCartney tracksuit gets even though it has been two years since the Olympic and Paralympic Games. I think this home Games will live in our hearts forever and the tracksuit, however old, will still be shining bright and stunning in front of any crowd. This was all so exciting and I was ushered into the courtyard to record a short interview while the crowd of a couple of hundred people all dressed to impress watched on! I felt very nervous and hoped that my words would be perfect. The flow just came out with my huge smile finishing it all off brilliantly!

'That's a wrap and you killed it!' said the young lady filming the interview. She was very impressed! I don't remember what I said but it must have been quite good because people kept mentioning that I had said the most amazing things!

We were then showed into St James's Palace and we had our own personal guide so didn't have to show any security to be allowed around the palace! I was awe with everything about the palace and the people working in there. There was gold everywhere which made the palace look so stunning!

Our personal guide showed us around the different rooms in the palace pointing out the gold on the walls and the artefacts from hundreds of years ago including the throne that the Queen sits on! The throne was made of pure gold! Amazing! It was absolutely incredible. 'You will be presenting the prizes after your speech in this room Stephanie'. WOW. Gold covered the walls. I was going to give other people awards in here in this amazing palace! Wow!

We went into a different room where a young lady did a short speech about how good the Duke of Edinburgh Awards had been for her then we were told to go into our specific rooms to do our own speeches and presentations. There were four people presenting prizes for each region: north, south, east and west. I was asked to do the west region! As we walked back into our rooms I was greeted by about two hundred students all sat around the room waiting patiently for my arrival. Their parents sat around them waiting to watch the presentation! The room was very large and could easily cope with the five hundred people situated in it now! Adrian and I were shown to our seats which were placed close to the door through which the Duke of Edinburgh would be leaving after his appearance! Adrian and I were told that we would be asked to stand by the door to be formally introduced to the Duke of Edinburgh after he had congratulated all of the Gold Award winners! We stood there patiently with me smiling happily to myself. We were given a five minute warning before the Duke of Edinburgh was going to arrive then closer to the time we were all told to stand up! My stomach fluttered with excitement!

Once he had entered the room only the winners of the gold awards were allowed to remain standing and the rest of us had to sit down and watch! The Duke of Edinburgh spoke to as many of the winners as he could as he made his way around the room. As he came around the last curve of the room Adrian and I were asked to stand up and move towards the door that the Duke of Edinburgh would be exiting from. When the Duke of Edinburgh reached us we were awarded a formal introduction to the Duke of Edinburgh! I had all ten Paralympic and World Championship medals around my neck and Adrian was carrying the Olympic Torch. We both felt so special! The Duke of Edinburgh shook Adrian's hand and questioned the torch and then noticed my glistening medals and, mesmerised, he asked me all about them.

'Are those medals heavy?' he asked.

My obvious reply was 'Yes would you like to hold them?'

'Oh gosh, they are heavy. Do they hurt your neck?'

'Oh yes!'

The Duke of Edinburgh was then ushered to the door as he had to visit all of the other rooms too! Just before he went out of the door he stopped, turned around to all of us and said 'Merry Christmas!' This was such a nice gesture but not something we had expected so everybody laughed!

Now was my turn. I did a short speech about my accomplishments where I specifically said that I was still chasing my dream, my gold medal, but that they were all amazing having reached their gold medals today so they were therefore inspiring me to win my gold medal! This got many gasps as they were in awe of me and therefore didn't think it was right for me to be wanting something that they were receiving today!

I was ushered into each of the four corners of the room where I was given an award to give to the winner when their name was been read out. There was a large amount of clapping after each name and this made the occasion very memorable! I spoke to each of the winners congratulating them for everything they had done to deserve this wonderful prize and asked them what they were going to concentrate on now. After all the awards were given out we were politely asked to make our way to the exit which we did but very slowly, appreciating every part of this special day! I was asked to sign a number of autographs and have pictures with the winners which I obviously loved! A lot of the winners were so inspired by what I had achieved and about London 2012 and what it had been like for me! I loved these questions as everyone was so interested in everything that had happened in London! It was an amazing Olympic and Paralympics Games which made everyone proud to be from Great Britain. We eventually made our way out of the palace with huge smiles on our faces.

The Duke of Edinburgh Awards was a wonderful finale to 2013! To be asked to present these amazing gold awards was an absolute honour. I hope that all children between fourteen and twenty-four do follow the Duke of Edinburgh charity and do achieve their awards! This is such a fantastic vessel in which kids are able to learn new life skills and to enjoy working hard to achieve their awards. I wish that I had taken up this challenge when I was younger as it creates such an incredible opportunity for everyone! I am a massive fan of the Duke of Edinburgh Awards charity and hope to remain an active volunteer in later dates when required!!

Thank you HRH Duke of Edinburgh!

I took some of my medals and the Olympic Torch to show all the other disabled riders to inspire them further. Everybody loved to hold them and have photos taken wearing the medals! I brought them back to the yard every week until everybody had seen them and touched them and had remembered their cameras!

One of the helpers at this RDA was Heather Marshall who was very inspired by my story and who asked if I could help to raise the profile of the RDA and of course I said yes. Heather is a very motivated person and when I told her I had MS and was a Paralympic swimmer she saw this as a perfect opportunity to get more funding for the Riding for the Disabled (RDA) charity that she was helping! Heather also told me about her best friend, Ros, who also has MS and would love to meet me. Heather has a horse called Tigs and she said if you come and meet Ros you can ride Tigs! Perfect! I get to ride another horse! I went to her yard a few days later and Heather introduced me to both Ros and Rodney, Ros's horse, and then to Tigs! Rodney pulled all sorts of faces at me trying to scare me but I just kissed him on the nose which really shocked him! Rodney was a gentle giant standing seventeen hands and two inches high which is very big! Rodney's best friend was Tigs who stood in the stable next to him. Tigs is a fifteen hands three inches coloured cob with a heart of gold! I gave them both a carrot and an apple so we are now friends for life and they know me as the treat girl! I rode Tigs who was very nice to ride then when I jumped off I struggled with standing as I do after racing in the pool. Heather ran off to get a chair for me! While sat in the chair Heather started riding. She looked so good on her horse and they worked together perfectly showing me all sorts of beautiful dressage moves. Tigs kept a close eye on me to make sure she didn't get too close to me sat in the middle of the riding school waiting for my legs to come back to me! In the end Heather, Tigs and I started jumping and went to different dressage competitions which I loved!

After doing the grooming and the tacking up and after sitting down for a while I started leading the horses around when other disabled riders were on board! After speaking with me Heather didn't let me run next to the horses when the riders were asked to trot but that was fair enough - I was scared that I would fall anyway!

Heather saw me as a perfect person to raise the profile of the Riding for the Disabled class at Widbrook and so set off with press releases for the newspaper about me and about how we needed to raise money to buy a new horse that the heavier riders could ride. Heather and I raised lots of money and lots of interest with loads of people coming to offer their help and support! I loved this because my misfortunes were giving something back to as many people as I possibly could! This was such a great feeling!

In the afternoons I helped year seven pupils from St Lawrence school to ride. These children had all different forms of special needs. One child couldn't speak and typed everything he wanted to say on a mini computer screen but he was truly inspired by my medals and the torch and he just kept smiling the whole time he was sat on the horses! Amazing! When I showed him my Paralympic medals he sent a text to his mum to get her to come to the stables asap which she did! They then had a photo with the boy, his mum, me and Chesney all together. It was such a lovely feeling helping so many people!

On Tigs I re-learned to ride properly with the help of Heather and Ros. Tigs was able to learn about my balance issues and on some occasions when my MS was being bad Tigs wouldn't go any faster than a walk in case I fell off as she felt that I was unstable on her back! What a super horse! Heather booked me in to compete on Tigs in a few shows and I won my first ever horse riding rosette! I was so excited. I made sure I had learned all my dressage moves even though we have somebody reading the instructions anyway: 'At A move into medium trot'. I loved this! I got a score of 57 which for my first ever test I was quite pleased with! I just need to work on this balance issue! I was so proud of my rosettes that I put them on Facebook! What a lovely achievement for me!

Heather invited Adrian and me to her house to meet Ken her husband who is a half-marathon runner and who, after meeting me was going to run the Bath half-marathon and raise money for the MS Society and the RDA (Riding for the Disabled) charity based in Bradford on Avon. Amazing! Ken made a comment that maybe one day he would push me sat in my wheelchair the whole thirteen plus miles for a half-marathon! This would definitely raise a lot of money! Ken came to Heather's yard once or twice when I was there and on one occasion he wanted a ride! This was so funny because although Ken had no balance issues he just kind of sat there legs straight, arms everywhere while Tigs tried to understand all the mixed messages Ken was giving to her! Tigs cantered around crazily and Heather, Ros and I were giggling away. It looked so funny. I am not sure Ken has quite copied the textbook for riding but it worked for him!

After many articles in the paper where we showed all our fund-raising exploits and our trips to different competitions trying to raise the profile of the RDA, Heather called me up one morning with some great news! A couple wanted to come to the yard to see the horses and to see me and chat about possible sponsorship! Wow!! Wonderful!

The Preeses arrived the following Monday and Heather and I had made Chesney and the other horses look as good as possible. The Preeses told us about their daughter who had gone on a family holiday skiing but who had unfortunately lost control of her skis on a ski run and had hit a tree. Unfortunately Jemima, their daughter, died from her injuries but they have created a charity, called Jemima's Gift, in honour of her life. This charity offers help to anyone wishing to do something special. The Preeses offered to buy a bigger horse for the RDA and to pay for its feed and insurance charges. Heather went out looking for this perfect horse and found him - Garfield! Garfield was brought to the yard and renamed Jemima's Gift as a show name and Jem as a stable name! What lovely people! From something bad came something so incredibly good!

CHAPTER 84
Spreading the Olympic Legacy

What is the Purpose of the Olympic Games?

The purpose of the modern Olympic Games is to promote peace and unity within the international community through the medium of sport.

The founder, Pierre de Coubertin, saw the Games as a way to bring political enemies together.

The modern Olympic Games were inspired by the ancient Olympic Games played during the Roman Empire. Those Games lasted for 1,200 years until about 400AD when the Games were banned by the Roman emperor at the time. After being involved in many battles, Pierre de Coubertin had the idea that sport could act as a way to build bridges between countries. In 1890 he formed the Union des Sociétés Francaises de Sports Athlétiques.

Four years later, de Coubertin proposed that the modern Olympic Games be created, and delegates representing nine countries agreed to his plan. The first modern Olympic Games were set for 1896 at the birthplace of the ancient Olympic Games: Athens. Pierre de Coubertin formed an international committee to organise the Games, and this grouping eventually became what is today known as the International Olympic Committee. Since that time, the Games has been shared around many countries with the goal of breaking down cultural barriers and bringing people together.

With thanks to: history1900s.about.com, olympics.sporting99.com

Legacy of the summer London 2012 Olympic Games

The future use of the Olympic Stadium and the park is the key to the legacy of the Games. The London 2012 Olympic Legacy is the longer-term benefits and effects of the planning, funding, building and staging of the Olympic and Paralympic Games. It is variously described as the following:

- Economic – supporting new jobs and skills, encouraging trade, inward investment and tourism. For example, 2012 apprenticeships in broadcasting companies including the BBC and ITV.
- Sporting – continuing elite success, development of more sports facilities and encouraging participation in schools sports and the wider community.
- Social and volunteering – inspiring others to volunteer and encouraging social change.
- Regeneration – reuse of venues, new homes, and improved transportation, in East London and at other sites across the UK. For example, the re-opening of the Olympic Park as the Queen Elizabeth Olympic Park in July 2013.
- Tourism – the Games' long-term benefits on London's and Britain's tourism industry.

The 2012 legacy is coordinated by the UK Government who appointed Lord Sebastian Coe as the legacy ambassador for London 2012.

The London bid for the 2012 Summer Olympic and Paralympic Games included bid chairman Lord Coe placing a pledge to use the events to inspire two million people to take up sport and physical activity at the heart of the bid. The term 'legacy' aims to ensure that no white elephants were created by the 2012 Summer Olympics and 2012 Summer Paralympics. The London Legacy Development Corporation is a mayoral development corporation responsible for the Olympic Park area.

The phrase 'white elephant' means a useless possession. Often, a white elephant is a burden in some way: large, difficult to store, or expensive to maintain. The story behind the phrase comes from the old traditions of Siam (Thailand). White elephants were very rare, so if the king gave one as a gift, it was an honour. However, the gift was a terrible burden to the person who received it. He had to feed and care for that elephant all throughout its long life!

Since the London 2012 Paralympic Games finished on 9 September 2012, the UK Government has unveiled an updated Legacy Plan. Its main points include:

- Funding for elite sport until Rio 2016.
- Investment to turn the Olympic site into the Queen Elizabeth Olympic Park.
- 20 major sporting events to UK by 2019, with more bids in progress.
- £1bn investment over the next five years in the Youth Sport Strategy, linking schools with sports clubs and encouraging sporting habits for life.
- Introduction of the School Games programme to boost school sport and county sport festivals.
- Continued funding for international Inspiration, the UK's international sports development programme, to 2014.

These initial plans seem to be working perfectly as from my point of view there seem to be more opportunities available, especially in the areas surrounding the Olympic Village including all the jobs in the Westfield shopping Centre!

The Olympic Games from my point of view is the pinnacle of any athlete's sporting career. The athlete trains for endless hours for the four years prior to the Olympic Games then comes to the Olympic Games along with many other athletes! It is a lovely feeling of togetherness when everyone is competing to be the best but also just to be a part of the same community or the same world. In Beijing the motto was: One world one dream! 'One World One Dream' fully reflects the essence and the universal values of the Olympic spirit of unity, friendship, progress and harmony. I love these four words as I think they say so much!! One World, One Dream!

Letter from HRH Prince Edward
3rd April 2012

Steph,

Hi. I understand that you would be happy to meet up with Prince Edward on the 3rd April. HRH is the new chancellor of the University and is President of the Paralympic Association and has asked if he could meet some of the Paralympians that train at the Bath University.

The programme is still being scheduled but it looks like he would like to meet you at 09.30 on the 3rd along with Ben Rushgrove, Katrina Hart and Tim Hollingsworth. Sophie Hamlish may also come but is heavy into exams at the moment and is not sure she can make it.

The idea would be to arrive at STV, the university, at around 09.30 and meet up with you and have a chat and possibly tea. I don't think it will be any longer than an hour at the most and the household officer will confirm the arrangements once she has talked them through with HRH.

We would need a short profile of you to send onto HRH in preparation of the visit; if you could send this through to me ASAP that would be appreciated.

I will let you know the final details as soon as they are confirmed.

Kind regards,

Ron
Ron Stewart
Sports Facilities Manager
Bath University

Thank you Ron and thank you to everyone else who works at Bath University's sports department. Thank you for wonderful opportunities such as meeting with HRH Prince Edward and thank you as well also for displaying an attention-grabbing banner congratulating me on winning four gold medals at the IPC World Championships.

Bath University have been a magnificent support for me with tweets and good luck wishes and I don't actually even represent Bath University when I race, although I wish I did. Maybe Bath University can take over Aquae Sulis? That would be amazing. All the employees at Bath University cheer me a merry welcome every morning at 05.30 when I wander in ready for my swim! They are such lovely people and I wish them all well.

Tim Hollingsworth (the Director of Sport & CEO for the BPA (British Paralympic Association)), a wonderful man with whom I have become good friends, was at this meeting and it was so nice to chat to Tim again. He is such a lovely person - always positive and always interested. He is an inspiring person to work with, as Adrian and I found out on a couple of other occasions when we were presenting awards for schools. I wish Tim the best of luck for everything he takes on in his life. To have you as a friend is heart-warming. Thank you.

Adrian was unable to come with me to meet HRH Prince Edward so I invited Charlie Head, who swims at Aquae Sulis with me. Charlie had written and produced a speech about me for his school which got him awarded an A grade! This inspired me so I decided he would be the perfect person to help with my medals. Charlie's parents were over the moon that I had asked him and they were eager to make Charlie look smart for his meeting with royalty! They decided to buy him a brand new school jacket and shirt and tie and he looked very dapper. They asked me what Charlie needed to do and I said that he should just smile and enjoy every minute! 'If there is a step can I have a little help but otherwise please just carry a number of medals and chat to everyone.'

Charlie did a perfect job and HRH Prince Edward was very impressed to see a young man carrying so many medals that he went straight to Charlie to chat. Their conversations went very well and I am certain he will always remember that moment.

Thank you, Bath University Sport Training village for offering us this wonderful opportunity.

Thank you also for displaying a stunning banner up in the entrance to the sports training village reading:

'Stephanie Millward four times IPC World Champion! 100m Freestyle, 100m Backstroke, 4x100m Freestyle Relay, 4x100m Medley Relay!'

This congratulatory banner was on show for a number of months and it made me feel so proud.

Stephanie Millward vs Multiple Sclerosis

Considering I may have MS for the rest of my life I have to learn to live with it and see it as a friend and not as an enemy. I need to know everything about it to see how to make it better and happier and to see what things make it sad or angry. The MS is now my friend and we can grow strong together. I call my MS a 'he' because men seem to be easier (generally) to understand than females! If I can't understand what MS is communicating to me, Adrian my guardian angel may be able to help me decipher his words. I know my MS hates heat and I know he hates humidity but I also know he (actually, probably more I) loves ice cream and lasagne.

Don't see the MS or other life altering illness as a negative bad thing. Try to think of these problems as opportunities. MS took a lot from me but in some ways it has given me wings so I can fly and see everything that I ever wanted to see! It has enabled me to meet lots of people and to help many others. MS has helped me to stop taking things for granted and to cherish everything that the world is giving us. I feel I have no boundaries with my kind heart. I love giving my heart to everyone to help make their life a more wonderful place to be. I am honest and genuine and wish to help everyone.

If I didn't have MS I fear I would only have thought of me. Now I have seen both sides: the abled and the disabled sides of life. As a result I am more humble, more experienced and more appreciative of opinions from others. As in maths, two negatives make a positive, so therefore every bad thing that happens could in some way be a very good thing. When Adrian asked me to marry him he also asked the MS knowing that it may be a lifelong thing. Adrian was so strong! The three of us Adrian, the MS and me are now in it forever. Together forever.

Offering inspiration

As you have read, I have been through quite a lot of mini tragedies throughout my life and that is why I feel the need to give back as much inspiration as I can on every occasion. If I change the thoughts or ideas of just one person that would be good enough. Just imagine if somebody hears my story and it drives them to become something they had only ever dreamed about but never realised was actually possible. Just imagine if somebody sends me an email in ten years' time that says, 'Thank you Stephanie, you helped me realise my dreams. I am now a GB basketball player' or 'I now work as a nurse helping people'. I try my hardest because that is what you always do. Thank you!'

What an inspiring thought. This kind of thought drives me on and makes me want to visit every school and go to all the events I possibly can. I love telling the children my story and giving them hope. Life is not meant to be easy but the fight is always worth it in the end and I am living proof that you sometimes get a second chance if you want it enough. Please grab that chance or that opportunity as best you can and become the superstar you have always wanted to be.

Circles of life!

My life seems to have been surrounded by strange circles.

China: I went to Shanghai, China, competing as the finale for my able-bodied perfect life and then returned to Beijing, China, as the opening debut appearance for Beijing 2008 Paralympic Games. This was my first return or circle.

Horse riding: I went horse riding once a week with friends of mine, Vicky and Sam Tye at Bradford on Avon's Widbrook Arabian Stud.

We absolutely loved riding and got excited after school when we went back to their house. Their mum, Maralyn, would plait our hair before we went to the stables. After giving up horse riding for swimming and school and after MS entered my life I returned with my friend Judy. We went to the same horse riding yard, Widbrook Arabian Stud, which I again loved. This was the second circle - a coincidental return to the same stables.

Swimming: I first started swimming in Jeddah, Saudi Arabia where my parents and the Saudi Sharks taught me how to swim. I have always been a quick learner and I remember the first time I ever swam butterfly was in a race which I won aged five! What a great start. We then left Saudi Arabia to live in the UK because of the Gulf War in 1990. My family moved to Manchester, then Swindon temporarily, then to our perfect home in Box, Wiltshire! Wherever we were living, I would train and compete, winning swimming trophies here there and everywhere – an affirming experience for a young girl. While I lived in Box I swam for Corsham ASC and then Bath Uni High Performance Centre (HPC). Swimming for me ended in 1999 when I fell ill with MS but then restarted again in 2006/7 when I wanted to lose weight. I then met Adrian and moved to Swansea HPC for a life as a Paralympic swimmer.

Saudi Arabia: After leaving Saudi Arabia in 1990 I never expected to go back again but swimming and the 2010 Commonwealth Games holding camp which was in Qatar, Saudi Arabia, brought me back! Incredible! When we arrived at the airport all the happy memories of my life in Jeddah came rushing back. I think I smiled the whole way through the camp. This is another circle I never expected to happen.

Bath University: When I was fourteen I was a very good swimmer, winning lots of county and regional medals, so my mum asked the people in charge of the brand new Olympic pool at Bath University if I could train there with their amazing Olympic swimmers (1996). Bath Uni agreed and I started training here but this unfortunately stopped on the 7th May 1999 due to my Multiple Sclerosis. I came back to train with Aquae Sulis at Bath University just after the London 2012 Paralympic Games in October 2012! The emotions on that first day were overwhelming with incredible sadness from the last time I had been at the university's swimming pool and also immense pride. I had fought through so much and finally I was back to somewhere I belonged!

Wiltshire's Swimmer of the Year: I had been awarded the Wiltshire's Swimmer of the year award twice before when I was able-bodied, and I won it again in 2013 after winning medals in London (2012) and in Montreal (2013). It was so strange seeing my name imprinted on the medals from so many years ago. Now I was such a different person but with the same name and the same love – swimming. Keep believing in your dreams always as you never know what might happen!

Box, Wiltshire. Back home at last: Box has always been a wonderful place to live. I first lived in a stunning house next to Box's recreation ground while I was growing up but unfortunately my parents divorced just after I fell ill with MS. This gorgeous house had to be sold quickly, and therefore for pennies, before my Mum and I moved to Chippenham to a smaller house and my Dad to Radstock. This all changed again when I moved to Swansea and my Dad moved to Lincoln. It has all changed again. My Mum moved to Devon to open her own business with her loving partner, Nick Woodall, who is an incredible person. People who deserve it are sent angels and I was sent Adrian and my Mum was sent Nick! All that pain was worth it in the end. Adrian and I moved to different rented properties when I moved back to Wiltshire/Bath but I felt very uneasy in all of them until, quite coincidentally, Mum spotted a flat in Box! Adrian and I had gone to visit our friends Sonia and Colin Bush. Colin said, 'Get in my car, let's go see this flat!' So we did! The owner was there too so he let us look at both the two flats which were available to rent. They were both beautiful. The views were vast and picturesque, the storage space was immense and the whole flat looked so welcoming.

Yeah! Count us in - we want to stay here in Box! I waited outside the estate agents the next day for about half an hour just so I was the first one in the line to put our names down for the flat. We moved in and both Adrian and I have felt so at home.

The owners of the flat, Nigel and Sarah, are excellent neighbours. They are the kindest people we have ever met. Nigel and I try to race to be the first to put all the bins out ready for collection on Monday morning and it is so funny in the morning as we drag everyone's bins out.

I have done my circle, leaving and then coming back to Box, and hopefully we will never leave. Box made me their Person of the Month in their newsletter and I gave out awards at the Box Revels yearly celebration. I was made to feel very welcome at their get to-gether which happens every Thursday between 10.00 and 12.00. I love being back in a place where I belong with lots of loving people around me surrounding me with happiness. My life is perfect. Since moving back to Box I have made friends with a lot of kind and self-less people. These people are the ones who do something solely to help someone else and not just to help themselves or to get money from it. I am surrounded by lovely people in my dream environment; I am home at last in a place where I truly belong.

Karen Grant: A number of years ago when I asked my mum to help me get a wheelchair she took me to a wheelchair unit where they measured me and gave me a suitable wheelchair. I hated it. I hated being in a wheelchair just because of the reason for it and so I decid-ed the wheelchair was only going to be used when necessary. Instead I would use the walls and other people's shoulders as my balance tools. The wheelchair was only used if I had to. I gave this wheel-chair back and bought my own when I started swimming again. On one occasion after London's Paralympics I was asked to re-open the wheelchair department. This was very strange as I remembered the first time I had been there very well. While I was opening this new initiative I met - Karen Grant - who was a lovely person. I left this event only to meet Karen again a long time later when I was invited to her children's school's sports day! We have been friends since and have gone to numerous events together.

Incidentally, Karen now does a lot of work with and for me and is a great support. She has two children Tom (11) and Rhys (7). They are such angels, always carrying my medals for me or taking a bucket round fetes trying to raise money for charities. They did a Katathon to raise sponsorship money to help me on my road to Rio. A Katathon is where a number of people - adults and children -show the audience a number of their moves (katas) that they had already learned. The karate master for the Patron Katathon was the director/chief instructor Nick Beaven. Nick Beaven runs his own martial arts school with many classes running during the week. (www.martialartleisure.com) Their mission statement is to promote a positive attitude towards health and fitness, to encourage people of all ability to exercise and feel welcome in a friendly and caring environment, to exemplify humility, self-control, integrity, courtesy and discipline. I loved the way they all worked together to be the very best they can be. I watched Tom (Karen's eldest son) complete and pass his black belt for karate and I was so impressed by how much he was enjoying it and how hard he worked for it. What a wonderful thing to learn. Nick Beaven was very kind and helpful, bringing people he knew to assist in this Katathon. The Katathon lasted five hours and it was fascinating to watch.

Karen has also taken on the role of 'Stephanie's agent' and does a lot of the chatting to people who want me to come to their events, either at their school or a presentation evening. This is so helpful as it makes my life that much easier. Thank you, Karen! Karen and I, with the help of a few other people, are organising a concert to raise money for the Amy Winehouse Foundation and myself, and for an army-related charity called 'Scotty's Little Soldiers' because Karen's husband, Oz, was in the army for twenty-two years!

On one occasion I was invited to go to London to attend the MS Societies Annual Awards in 2012 and to give out some awards which Adrian and I did. The meal was delicious and the table I was sitting at meant I met some incredible people. When Kate Silverton, the BBC news presenter who often presents for the MS Society, started reading out who had won MS inspiration of the year award I opened my mouth in awe...

'...at fifteen she was British record holder, all excited and training for Sydney Olympics in the year 2000. But then instead of going to Sydney she went blind and was paralysed...'

I smiled! That was my life and my MS story! I had indeed won MS Society's MS inspiration of the year! What an honour. I went on stage and was awarded a beautiful trophy which I was very proud of as I didn't expect it.

I gave out another award and when the presentation part was over I started chatting to everyone. What an evening it turned out to be. I met a lovely woman on this event and she is like a goddess. Her name is Tessa Lush - what a wonderful name. Tessa is incredible and she is an amazing support. Tessa couldn't believe that I didn't have any sponsors!

I was asked to do the introduction and instruction parts of Sym-Trac which I love watching back. We had a wonderful day of filming at Corsham's Springfield Centre which was great fun. Thank you so much, Tessa. It is so heart-warming that I have so many wonderful, amazing friends now. Finding friends like these has been inspirational for me.

One great friend of mine lives in London and is a truly fantastic compere for balls or any other charity fundraisers. This wonderful man's name is Roger Dakin and he has connections with just about everybody! Roger raises money for all sorts of charities and he has helped me. What an exceptional man! Another charity that I am personally connected with is Bags4Sport which is owned by Andy Trusler. Andy was the one who invited me to go to London with him to meet Roger in the first place. Bags4Sport is a charity that raises money for up-and-coming young sports people. I was awarded £500 to help with my costs. Through Andrew Trusler I also met Gordon Straker, an incredible estate agent, who has been such a support as well.

While in London, Roger invited me to stand in front of the large roomful of business men in suits at a business lunch, where he asked me loads of questions about my life and about the medals I had won. I stood there in my GB kit with my five Paralympic and five World Championships medals around my neck. The crowd were quiet when I said I had gone blind and was paralysed and how I employed someone to teach me how to stand. Everyone had been listening but one amazing man got back in touch with me after the meeting saying that he would like to help me with sponsorship. Simon Millar from Monopoly Network (monopolynetwork.co.uk) held a ball where he raised loads of money which he split equally between me and another charity, Scotty's Little Soldiers (www.scottyslittlesoldiers.co.uk). We went to a lunch in London where Adrian and I met loads of interesting people. Scotty's Little Soldiers and I were each awarded just over £13,000 to help with, in my case, the road to Rio! What an amazing company and what an incredible man! Thank you, Simon!

I love going to different venues and different events because I love seeing the smile on people's faces. Whenever people see the Olympic Torch or the Paralympic medals they are truly awe-struck. I try my hardest to inspire everyone I meet.

'They are so heavy!' is the reply I got every time someone holds my trophies. 'I didn't think they would be this heavy!'

One of my absolute greatest supports is Pak from the Hong Kong House Chinese Takeaway which is situated in Corsham. Pak came to my Freedom of Corsham celebration and gave me a lovely bouquet of flowers and has always given me good luck wishes for the Paralympics in Beijing and London! Pak has photos of him and me up on the wall in his Chinese takeaway and this photo is just under the one of the Queen. I feel so honoured to have this amazing support - thank you Pak. Whenever I go to pick up my Chinese meal there is always someone there who enjoys seeing the medals and Olympic Torch. I love his Chinese and I love his wonderful support.

What have I learned?

I am seeing a psychologist at the moment and she asked me one question, 'What did you lose through MS when you had the perfect life training for Sydney?'

EVERYTHING, was my reply, everything. I lost my eyesight, I lost my ability to walk, I lost the control we all expect of our bladder and bowel, and I lost my memory, my dogs and some friends. My parents got divorced, I lost my future career and my confidence and my independence. But the one thing that I could never lose was my dream, that Olympic gold medal. The thing inside my heart that could never be taken away. Look at the amazing life stories of Muhammad Ali, Gandhi, Sylvester Stallone and Pinocchio and see how they defeated adversity to achieve their dream. These are in my opinion, the superstars I have been following. They are my heroes! A lot of people ask me who my hero in the sporting world is and I say I don't really have one (although Mark Foster has always been inspirational to me!). The reason I don't have one is because it is almost a way of limiting my chances. I want the opportunity to be the best I can be for me and I try not to be as good as any person in particular.

Another question I am often asked is, 'What time did you swim today?' I want to swim as fast as I can swim. Putting a time on a swim is a way of slowing you down or limiting your chances. Believe the impossible and anything is possible! Also, open your eyes to every new opportunity. If one door closes another one will open, somewhere. Be open and excited about any change. If you lose your job look at it as a good thing because now you can strive for something else you enjoy doing. Life is for living.

I lost that easy, perfect life to make or to turn me into a nicer, stronger person and to open up opportunities there was no way I would have been offered otherwise: winning numerous Paralympic medals; Carrying the Olympic Torch; presenting awards at the Duke of Edinburgh Awards; Winning the MS Societies Inspiration of the Year; meeting Novartis and Tessa Lush! I have experienced blindness, paralysis, heartbreak but then pure absolute love, devotion and marriage! I am a lucky, lucky person!

If there is a wall in your way stopping your path look for other ways to go around the wall, over the wall or under it! Make life fun and exciting as remember that every day is a new page in a new chapter of your book and you are the author so you are in charge. You can do anything you want to!

Always look up! This world is one amazing place to be! Spread happiness! Smile!

CHAPTER 85

Plans for the Future

Plans for the future? What am I meant to say? I hope I complete all my dreams and that my ambition kills all the bits of regret I was feeling after both the Sydney and Beijing Olympic Games where I didn't do as well as I had wanted to. I do hope this but most of all I hope I am happy and I hope the rest of my family are happy too. Dreams are wonderful but a lot of the time they are only a fantasy and therefore they will just live when we are sleeping or when we are day dreaming. Most dreams need to be reassessed and turned into something a little easier to reach. I mean, every single one of us would love to win the lottery but the likelihood of winning it is not very high and perhaps the two pound sterling we spend is a waste of our money but maybe it is a way of keeping our dreams alive. With swimming it is a little more about believing. If you believe you can do something you are more likely to be able to achieve it because if you do not believe in yourself there is no way you will get to where you wish to be.

My life has been a lot to do with belief and desire. I wanted to be the best but my dreams were taken away from me and instead replaced by pain and tears, by an incurable illness I will probably have for the rest of my life. I am not sure what I did to deserve this but this uncertainty has been strengthened by the belief I have in myself to swim well and to keep fighting. Adrian has been my angel, standing by my side always whispering words of wisdom and psychologically coaching me to reach my dreams. Everything I have ever desired is getting closer and the tear-stained cheeks have been replaced by a vividly refreshing pink and the frown by the huge welcoming smile. My life has turned into a new chapter and therefore has a new subject and includes more exciting items. I look forward to every day and to opening every page of my story. My life has been hard but all the harsh times I have experienced and all the things that I have learned have made me a wiser and better person. I believe now that I deserve the life I am living and I also know that I am the person who can realise her dreams and who can enjoy every day as a child does with fresh attention and lively ideas. I am lucky I have been given a second chance!

MS - My war

An incurable illness, no cure no treatment
A debilitating disease – a fight, my war
Why does my life hurt me so much?
When will all the pain be gone?

I am a survivor, but I want to die
I am a fighter but I want to quit
A large battle that I am now loosing
An endless war, I cannot win

Look in the mirror see a smile on your face
Look inside see a life full of pain
MS is invisible, I can disguise my health
MS destroys lives, can't hide from myself.

I try to look up but my life is declining
I stare at the stars but my life is still sliding
Who's going to help me rid my life of the pain?
Who can I rely on to relight my life flame?

We are waiting for a life
But will a cure ever be found?
My heart has been broken, leaving two halves
The cure, my lifesaver, will rebind my heart.

I will then be able to realise my dreams
The future fears will all be gone
The pain will be tied down and controlled
The torturing disease locked up behind bars.

MS breaks a thousand hearts
Heart and feelings, Hopes and dreams
The cure will end my life of worries
When will that special second ever be?

I am a survivor, I can't fade away
I am a fighter so I will not give in
A large battle that I will not lose
An endless war, I have to win.

Stephanie Millward Copyright 2000

We, as a family have got through something that I wouldn't wish on anyone else. It was hard and at times I thought that we weren't going to make it. I was fighting this almost hidden battle. The legs weren't working properly and the eyes had just about given up but with strength and determination we held on to the last millimetres of hope and strength. I used my family's words as stepping stones to get better and stronger. They were trying to get a perfect life for themselves because they had watched their daughter, or sister lose her near-perfect world. They were fighting to get their lives perfect for me, to offer their support that way. If they were happy I can be happy for them and get strength that way when the times were hard. MS ripped me into a million pieces but my family and close friends have started to put the jigsaw pieces back together and eventually I am certain everything will be fixed! I didn't do anything wrong and neither did my family so this war that we are fighting must have a reason, a light, a star at the end!

Four times world champion.
Five times London Paralympic Games medallist.
Olympic Torchbearer.
MS Hero?!
My MS war is in my eyes already WON!

My story is not about a girl who lost her career, her health, her dad, her dog and her friend but instead is about a young lady who was walking through a dark tunnel, eventually reaching the light at the end and meeting her guardian angel, her partner for life - the fairytale story. My story is a little harsher than other fairy stories but it is still about reaching all the goals of the younger girl and even of realising all her dreams. It is a story about hope and about inspiration even through the dark times. It is a book about becoming the person you have always dreamed about becoming. A shattered perfection rebuilt to enable the light to reflect again. The end to one of those stunning rainbows.

This is a story about my life and I hope it makes you smile and feel strong!
Keep believing and keep dreaming!

My love, always!
Stephanie

ACKNOWLEDGEMENTS

Thank you to everyone who helped me come to terms with a currently incurable disease of my central nervous system Multiple Sclerosis and for helping me to fight to be the best at my chosen field in life as a Paralympic swimmer. I couldn't have done it without your encouragement and your support. Thank you so much for everything you have done for me!

My Mum Linda Millward (always there for me!)
My Husband Adrian Millward-McHugh (my angel)
My Dad Christopher Michael Millward
My Brother Paul Millward
My Sister Kristy Millward
My Brother Nicholas Millward
My Mum's partner Nick Woodall
My Dad's wife Diana Millward
Paul's wife Kerry Millward
Kristy's husband Mike Perkins
Dale Pollard & Alison McHugh
Tyrone & Tyson Pollard
Daren Henry& Andrea McHugh & Liam Henry
John & Joan McHugh
Matt & Sarah Leighton-Fry
Neil Harris & Ibby Wallace
Peter & Linda Woodgate
Paul Langely (incredible caring man)

Stephen Brown (makes dvds for me! Amazing support)
Alistair & Jeannie Hignell (incredible)
Colin & Sonia Bush (always there for Adrian & me.
    Amazing friends)
Carl & Ryan Bush
Ken & Heather Marshall (superstars)
Andrew Desmond (world's best photographer)
Ros Dobson
Mike & Caroline Cox (amazing people)
My Swimming Coaches: Peggy Tanner, Julia Airlie, Ian Turner,
    David Lyles, Martin Mosey, Stephen Fivash, John Dougall
    & Billy Pye
Robert James
Oliver Holt & family
Roger Dakin
Margaret Carey
Tom & Rhys Grant (& their Dad Oz)
Maddy Elliot & her family!
Colin Bush Machinery
Monopoly Network
Martin & Sylvia Howland
Amy (Wazzy!) Howland
Clare Wilson
Vanessa & Nicole
Alice Kemp, Janet Anderson-Mackenzie
Peter Hassel (Swimming Times)
Dave Stone
Caroline Petrinolis & her wonderful daughters
Fran O'Connor (Franakins!)
Gemma Almond (incredible friend)
Ellie Simmonds (the one & only)
Will Walder (amazing man)
Daryl, Amy & Joe Jelineck
Stuart Gibbs
Tessa Lush

Gail Seviour
Andy Milton
Andy Trusler (Bags4sport)
Natalie Brown
Shaha Shah
Catherine Weatherburn
Bill & Silke Moore & the Mutual Support Crew
Chris Leigh (an amazing Facebook & twitter support!)
Alison Glower Negata (physio)
Gary Evan (Greatwood)
Nick Beaven (martial arts)
Vix Edwards (Twitter friend!)
Corsham Town Council
Wiltshire Council
Swansea Council
Swansea Police Force

Two very important people I wish to thank are Jess Nel and Karen Grant. Jess has helped me write a couple of chapters and has edited my book. Jess is an incredible person full of charm and virtue. She tried to complete everything as well as she could!

Karen has been a huge support acting as my agent and becoming an incredible friend for life! We have visited places expecting nothing and coming out with huge smiles on our faces! Karen you are an angel in disguise always working hard to make sure that everything you can do you will do! Thank you so much for everything.